GALEN

GALEN

By Allan Gilbreath

Galen

Published by
Kerlak Enterprises, Inc.
Kerlak Publishing
Memphis, TN
www.kerlak.com

ISBN: 0-9788777-0-5
ISBN 13:978-0-9788777-0-5
Library of Congress Control Number: 97-97097
First Printing 1997
Second Printing 1998
Third Printing 2006

Special thanks to Delois and Celeste for all the encouragement and assistance.

This book is printed on acid free paper.

Printed in the United States of America

Galen casually strolled between the marble monuments to lives now over. This close to the water, coffins couldn't be placed in the ground so this city of the dead came into being. As he passed families placing flowers and paying their respects, he fought the urge to smirk at their tears. At least, he was honest about why he killed. While he was sure that the family as a whole missed their dearly departed, he was also sure that members were secretly happy at being relieved of their caregiver duties. Others may miss the grandfather, but they seemed to be enjoying the inheritance. Already bored with the petty concerns of humans, Galen continued his quiet exploration.

One crypt in particular captured his attention. The angel adorning the front had actually been carved in the likeness of the woman who laid at rest here. In the failing light of dusk, the dimming sunlight cast a reddish glow over the aged marble. Galen found the trick of the light both amusing

1

and appropriate. He had known her well enough to kill her.

They had traveled together for decades. It would be inaccurate to have called them lovers. They may have loved being together, but neither of them had any illusion about themselves and their ultimate fates. She had already begun to suffer from chronological fatigue when they met. Galen's mental prowess and raw savagery had been enough to revive her interest in continued existence for a while. In the end, Galen ended her boredom and placed her here.

To be perfectly honest, he couldn't even remember her name. At this point, the dead held place of reverence for him. The death of others merely allowed him to continue to cheat time. He had actually come to admire the exquisite marble work of her likeness.

Time and nature had already done their work. The fine details had been worn away and moss had grown into the fine cracks. The last time he stood here, the stonework literally shone. He placed his hands on the rusted fence. Everything around him seemed to fade so quickly. She had warned him that this would be the first sign of the fatigue. He stared into the still fierce eyes of the statue. His time hadn't come yet. A faint purple glow appeared on the carved face as a ray of sunlight reflected from his ring. He looked down at the royal purple stone. In spite of its great age, neither the stone nor the gold that held it showed any sign of falling victim to the passing of ages.

As long as that ring resisted fading into dust, so would he. Galen smiled at his own bravado in the face of faded stonework. Time may overcome everything eventually, but it would have to wait for him. The human world grew more interesting by the day and he had no intention of missing the show.

He would adapt and continue. Galen gave the marble face one last look then turned and walked away. He would not return.

CHAPTER ONE

He slowly rubbed his hands together as he watched her walk into the light. An archaic ring stood out as a dark stain against his hand in the darkness. The reflecting fog eddying around her well-formed body was artwork in motion. He pressed his hands to his lips as if praying and exhaled slowly. He enjoyed her performance like a fine wine. A smile moved slowly across his face like rain across parched land. His eyes focused intently on the curves of her body and his thoughts focused on the pleasure she would bring him tonight. From his vantage point on the cross member of the bridge twenty feet above the pavement, he could sense that all the pieces of his game had fallen into place.

As if on cue, the rear door of the Cadillac below opened and stood in silent invitation. The woman stepped expectantly towards the beckoning door. She wrapped her arms around herself as the chill in the air made itself known. She shivered slightly with excitement as well as the cold. This was better than she could have hoped. The mystery of it all began to thrill her. Alone, on a deserted bridge, in the middle of nowhere, just like in all those old movies.

The night air seemed to be getting colder as she looked into the backseat. Surprisingly, there was no one there, instead, laid out across the seat lay a beautiful full length fur coat. The cold continued to intensify as she stroked her hand slowly across the fur. It felt so good, cool, and soft to the touch as only a very expensive fur could feel. She carefully pulled the coat from the car and with one last stroke slipped into it. A big hug across the arms and a little swirl finished the inspection.

"Galen?" She asked over the sound of the lapping water. "Galen, where are you?" Only fog moved across the lights from the vehicles. "Galen, this is fantastic. Where are you? I have something for you." The last few words dropped off into a husky whisper.

Another minute of the slowly moving fog and silence passed as her mood changed from adoration to concern. There was no one to be seen as she looked around. A quick glance through the car door revealed only an empty backseat.

He watched as she discovered the coat. He could feel the fur under her fingers as she stroked it. He felt its cool embrace as she slipped into it. His eyes closed in pleasure as he tasted the change of her mood. He felt the quickening of her pulse as his own pulse rose to match. The sensations had grown almost more than he could bear as he whispered "Now," into the night air.

She jumped when she saw a movement in the Cadillac. Someone rose up from the floorboard of the front seat. Her heart pounded with both fear and relief as she attempted to recover her composure. This was supposed to be her fantasy and she should be in control. The anticipation, mixed with the new element of suspense, had her breath coming hard. Each breath proved to be an event magnificently demonstrated by her full breasts rising and falling. The nipples already peaked by the chill and much more. They clearly attempted to press through the thin cloth confining them.

The passenger side door opened. A light breeze touched her face as if to announce the arrival. The figure slowly began to stand and straighten to its full height. The fog diffused light turned this simple act into a surrealistic ballet of shadow and movement.

She gasped and inhaled deeply. She had unconsciously been holding her breath for the last few moments. This was the most incredible thing that had ever happened to her. The expression on her face bore witness to her feelings. She slowly took a step towards this enigmatic figure before her. As her foot touched down she became enveloped in cold. Not the cold of the night, but a cold that seemed to grip her very flesh and blood. Something had gone very wrong. The sound of a deep inhale reached her. She felt her knees begin to weaken. Her feet defied the impulse to run. Her breath caught as the figure raised its hands.

"My God, what's wrong with me? What's happening?" She cried as she fought back against the rising panic. "What are you doing to me?"

He leaned dangerously forward on the cross beam above the figures bathed in fog below. His eyes betrayed the predatory nature of the seduction he had orchestrated. The smell of sex, surprise, and now fear emanating from the woman intoxicated him. He savored each and every moment of the bizarre scene. Every nerve sang out under the strain. Every muscle tightened and twisted like steel springs pushed to the bursting point. "Not yet," he told himself with grim determination. "The best is yet to come."

As if some invisible string had been pulled from above, the figure stepped from behind the car door and into the ghostly light. Her primal scream tore into the night. She became filled with the knowledge that the relationship to be explored here tonight was not one of man and woman, but one of predator and prey. The cold intensified as she looked into those cat-like eyes. The returned stare told her there was no one to plead with, no one to listen to her beg for life, so she screamed again.

"Now to finish this!" The cry of triumph sang out from the darkness above the cars. He leapt to his feet and looked to the end of the bridge where she had entered from the road. At the second scream, a set of headlights appeared. He smiled tightly. As if speaking an arcane incantation, he beckoned, "Come on now, it's your turn. Come now, you have your part to play." Smugness washed his face as he heard the awaited car approach.

Steve hadn't had a good week. First, his girlfriend broke up with him. She won't tell him what's wrong, but he knows it is that new guy he's seen her with. This morning he got this note saying she was sorry and had been wrong. He went out to see her and the crazy bitch threw some kind of tantrum. She screamed at him. She even called him a jealous pig and a liar. Well, nobody was going to call him a pig and a liar and get away with it. He decided to follow her out this evening and when he could get his hands on this new boyfriend he was going to give him a good old-fashioned ass-whipping. That'd show her how he really felt.

Now, Steve knew she had lost her mind. She had driven all the way out of town in the fog and now she had parked in the middle of a bridge, in the middle of the night. He reached over and picked up the last beer out of a twelve pack. He popped the top and raised the can to his lips. He nearly choked when the scream hit him like a shock wave.

"What the hell?" He blurted out as he looked out across the bridge. It didn't do much good in the fog. The second scream hit as the engine of the 76' Camaro roared to life. The clutch, the gas, then the tires sent up a shower of gravel as he hit the lights. Steve could see her backing away from someone. The guy stood in the middle of the road and walked slowly towards her. The figure turned and stared into his headlights. Steve felt mesmerized for a moment. His eyes locked with those strange orbs reflecting back red like some kind of nocturnal animal. Fear finally broke the spell and Steve slammed on the brakes. The moist pavement wouldn't allow the tires to grip. The momentum caused the Camaro to veer towards the parked Cadillac. At the last moment, Steve braced for the impact. His knuckles went white on the steering wheel as he pressed the brake to the floor in desperation.

Steve's head bounced off the top of the steering wheel as bones snapped and metal twisted at the front of the car. The engine stalled. He didn't care as he leaned back and moaned. He rubbed his forehead and moaned again. The car door opened and Steve got out painfully. He leaned against the side of the Camaro and shook his head from side to side. He looked to the front of the car as the panic began to set in.

"Oh no, God no! I didn't want to kill the guy. No, no, no." Steve's voice trailed off. He looked past the hood at the ground. It was worse than he could have imagined. The guy appeared to have exploded. As Steve got closer, the odor hit him. He recoiled at the stench. With his shirt bunched up in front of him, held over his mouth, Steve took another look. Nothing made sense. This guy should be bleeding all over the place not just kind of oozing. Like rotten meat in advanced decay, the stench became overpowering. The mottled and pallid skin had literally burst apart. It looked more like he ran over a month old corpse than a man who was just standing in the middle of the road. Steve stepped back remembering he was here because of her.

"Jean, what the hell is going on here?" He asked angrily. There was no answer. "Jean, dammit! I'm talking to you."

She just stood there at the side of the bridge next to the ironwork staring up into the fog. Steve walked over and grabbed her by the shoulders and shook her until she looked at him.

Everything had been going perfectly. Nothing was supposed to go wrong. She should not be able to move. The revenant must have been losing its powers. After all, it had been with him for almost six months now and they really didn't last much longer than that. Now, he would have to find and train another one. With all the remorse of losing a not so favorite pet, he retrained his focus on her again. She would stay. His powers had not weakened. He inhaled again deeply. That fool below was going to pay for this unexpected change in tonight's orchestration. Slowly, gracefully, he stretched his arms out and flexed like a great cat. He had enough of foreplay. It was time to finish this. It was time to feed.

"Hello."

Steve spun at the cultured word that dropped out of the swirling mist. He didn't hear the stranger drop from the beam above to the gleaming pavement. Steve looked him over, quickly sizing him up. About average, Steve was going to enjoy a fight tonight.

He never saw the slap coming. It ripped across the side of his face, spinning him almost backwards. Steve tasted blood in his mouth. First came a wave of fear, then the cold hit as he looked back at his attacker. Steve could see some kind of steam rising off his own body and floating over to him. His knees began to feel weak.

Steve cried out "NO!" in defiance and launched himself at the approaching figure. He lashed out with a massive right hook that flew by its target harmlessly. The same results happened with the left hook. Two more punches agonizingly missed by fractions of an inch. Steve tired rapidly as the cold wrapped around him, condensation frosting his hair. One last desperate lunge and he managed to get his hand on that bastard's shirt. All he felt was a light tap at his wrist and a slap above his eye. The impacts wouldn't have harmed a small child, yet the world spun around him once and fell in on him with that one word mocking him.

The man crumpled in front of him. The stranger could now see the object of his desire. Humans could be so simple to handle. Touch them just right and they collapse like rag dolls thrown from their stands. He casually stepped over the shallowly breathing body.

"You will stay right here until I am ready for you, won't you? Of course you will."

Steve couldn't answer as the stranger stepped over him and then away.

"Thank you my dear for a magnificent evening. I have had a wonderful time." The stranger said casually. "Tonight has been more than I could have ever hoped and just look at you, you look ravishing."

He gingerly took her hands in his and caressed them gently. He slowly massaged his way to her wrists. His fingers worked in ever increasing circles. The muscles of her forearms didn't attempt any form of resistance to his advance. The biceps gave in just as easily. Her flesh submitted instantly to the questing fingers. She sighed deeply when the fingers and the accompanying sensations reached her shoulders. She would have collapsed had her legs obeyed her as he traced the lines of her silk blouse under the coat. With obvious delight, he slid the blouse and coat off her shoulders, freeing her breasts to the night air and pinning her arms to her sides. A husky moan escaped her as her nipples brushed across his cotton shirt.

She had seen everything. She had heard everything. She simply couldn't cry out. She couldn't run. All she could do was watch Galen leave Steve on the ground like a broken doll and come to her. Her skin thrilled to Galen's touch. Strangely, she couldn't feel any warmth from him. Certainly, anyone at this point should feel a little warm. She could no longer feel the cold as he held her shoulders. Her body completely betrayed her when he caressed her breasts. They wanted more.

Galen lightly kissed her on the neck. The sensation ran through her like liquid lightning. He kissed her again on the neck, this time more insistently. Even though she would have melted to the ground, if that had been allowed, she could feel no warmth in the kiss. He lifted his head slightly. If she could have seen his face she would have seen the ivory teeth glinting in the light. Galen inhaled deeply as if trying to take in all the air about them. He thrilled to the sensation of her warmth. He almost wished that this could continue a bit long, but he had gone too far to stop now. He had to have what he needed and he had to have it now.

She felt the pressure, then the penetration of her skin. Surprised at how little pain she felt, she focused on the flood of heat. The rush of heat left her body and flooded into his as every inch of her being screamed out in bizarre sensations. The pressure at her neck was sensual and irresistible. She moaned loudly and pressed her body up against his. Her breasts cried out for contact with his chest. She began to lose consciousness. She couldn't feel her legs any more. Her arms hung limply at her side. It was as if she were deflating and drifting away at the same time. All she could remember was that she planned to give him something, but she couldn't remember what it was.

Chapter Two

Maggie looked tired as she got out of what could best be described as what remained of a weather beaten, red car. It had been a long day. She jiggled the key in the door of the townhouse. The door had been recently painted the same uninspired blue as the other hundred front doors in the complex. She lived in the second row of buildings, so she wouldn't have to put up with a lot of the noise from the main road out front. That was why she rented this one, that and the fact this was where she lived five years ago, before she had gotten married.

The sight that greeted her didn't do much to cheer her up. Moving boxes remained stacked everywhere. She stepped over packing material and wads of newspaper to the secondhand couch. Doing her best imitation of that commercial, she flopped over backwards landing heavily on the cushions.

"Welcome home, Maggie DeVane. Remember, this is the first day of the rest of your life." She

14

remarked with as much mockery as she could muster.

At least ten minutes passed before she even attempted to kick off her shoes. Toes against the heel of the shoe, a little grunt, followed by a small push and a tremendous moan of relief completed the action. She closed her eyes and breathed slowly as she replayed the day on the inside of her eyelids.

It began with sunlight. Actually, it began with too much sunlight. During the night the shade had rolled up leaving her exposed to this unwelcome invasion before the alarm clock had its chance. Maybe the shade and the alarm clock had conspired against her. No sooner than she had gotten out of that comfortable bed, walked across that cold floor, pulled that traitorous shade back down, and returned to the edge of the still warm mattress than the blasted alarm clock began that shrill chirp that grabbed you by the spine and made sleep impossible.

The next surprise of her new townhouse proved to be the shower. After stumbling around the bedroom, half looking through the boxes, half trying to go back to sleep, she finally discovered the hidden towels. With her prize slung over a shoulder, she poorly navigated the doorways and made it to the bath. Maggie, never much of a morning person, really didn't feel like rising to the challenge now presented by a new home and the maze of unpacked boxes. She managed to get the tap running in the tub. After several attempts to get the temperature just right she lifted the handle that started the shower. A disappointing gurgle and a thin spray of water began. The showerhead had become almost completely clogged. It amazed her to learn what could be accomplished with a tub, a washcloth, and a bad attitude.

Finding her work clothes, panty hose, etc. in different boxes scattered throughout the place provided a unique form of intellectual stimulation. After a quest that rivaled the Holy Grail for a matching pair of shoes, a cup of coffee would have been nice. She managed to find the cup, the coffee, and even the decanter, but no coffee machine. Maggie managed to find a way to force the cup into her purse on the way out the door to work.

The office hadn't changed in the five years she had been away. While a few new faces wandered by, mostly she saw a lot of old familiar ones. This gave her a very reassuring feeling. She was happy to see old Mr. Morley was still with the firm. The sight of the small spare tire and the bald head of the man who had to be seventy if he was a day meant that there was a cup of coffee brewing in here somewhere. Maggie thought Morley would prefer coffee to breathing. He always had a cup working.

Happy to show her around, a few of the old familiar faces finally showed her to her desk. In a tongue-in-cheek ceremony, they presented her with a small potted plant and her old nameplate, Ms. Margaret DeVane, CPA. The rest of the morning was spent gossiping, and getting acclimated to the old routine. By late afternoon, the job felt the same as it had always been. Now, the routine was comfortable, not the tedium she had felt before. With all the changes in her life lately, it was nice to be back in familiar territory.

The clock on the far wall had begun to creep up on five o'clock when she saw another familiar face, Michael Lawson going from desk to desk. Maggie immediately recognized the look on his face. Nothing ever changed, well, at least not Michael. He must have a "big" client ready to sign up. Every time he pulled a large client in he liked to put on a big "just one happy family" social event. The bigger the client, the bigger the party he threw. Five years really hadn't changed Michael much. About 5'7" and 250 lbs, he still moved around easily. He didn't have that "heavy" look most men his size moved with. Very well dressed, the red paisley tie had been smartly set off with a monogrammed gold tie clip. The white shirt still looked pressed even after a busy workday. The dark blue pinstripe suit had been obviously tailored to make his bulk look its best. He was a salesman of the most deadly kind. He didn't look like one.

"Maggie." He said as he stepped up to her desk smiling.

"Yes, Michael. What can I do for you?" She smiled back.

"Well, Maggie, first of all, I would like to say how happy I am to see you back with us. Now, maybe we'll get a little work done around here."

"Well, Michael, first of all, I would like to say how happy I am to be back at work here," she leaned back and did her best to imitate his practiced rolling tones, "and, yes, we might even get a little work done." Maggie hadn't had much fun the last couple of years and it felt good to play a little bit.

Without missing a beat, Michael continued, "Secondly, I'm giving a little get together tomorrow night at O'Brian's for the office and our new client." His voice now deepening, "but of course, a new international client is only the pretense. The true reason is to welcome you home and show you how we really feel about you." He finished with a wink.

Maggie answered in what may have been the worst Hungarian mixed with British accent ever attempted, "Well dahhhhlink, just how do you feel about me?"

Before Michael could answer the speaker on the phone came to life and a young male voice broke in. "Hey Maggie, it's great to have you back and all that, but it's 5:00 and I need to run backups on the systems. So, can you two try out for Masterpiece Theater after you log out."

Maggie reached for the phone console and pressed a button and spoke loudly at it. "Sorry, Rob, I'm logging out now. Hey, you gonna go tomorrow night?"

The voice on the speaker came back, "O'Brian's always taste better when it's on Mike's credit card."

Michael leaned slowly over to the phone and in a deadpan voice quipped, "Rob, you're coming.

18

Good. Oh, by the way, did I mention that it will be the all-you-can-eat tripe and buttermilk buffet."

"Boy, you really know how to impress the clients." The voice replied very flatly.

After taking a moment to get the silly grin off her face and to make a few swift keystrokes she turned to Michael with a disdainful look and asked, "So, who's the new client we're all supposed to impress?"

"He's an image consultant from Europe. He's been over here for five or six years, off and on. He said he liked it over here and needed a "reputable firm" to look after his affairs. He travels around helping the new rich act and look like old money. He apparently makes a very good living at it." Michael talked with his hands. His words and movements danced perfectly in synch.

"Oh lovely, dinner out with the troops and a pompous stuffed shirt from Europe. How can I possibly refuse?" Maggie said smiling broadly. With Michael doing the company's huckstering, Morley making coffee, and Rob still whining about the "backups" it felt like no time had passed at all.

Maggie slowly smiled as she completed her review of her first day back and gathered up enough strength to sit up and restart the dreaded process of unpacking. After clearing through a couple of the large boxes and carrying the packing out to the dumpster, the place started to shape up. She found a repair notice on the sink in the bathroom stating that maintenance had fixed the shower. The towels and everything else she needed for the bathroom had now been found and put away in a far more convenient location. Maggie decided to let a bath take her away.

Her hair still wet, Maggie sat down on the couch. She rubbed the back of her head with the towel draped over her shoulders. She began sorting through the contents of a large cardboard box sitting on the table in front of her. She slowly unwrapped gnomes, glassware and other mementos.

Carefully, she sorted them out on the plain wooden coffee table. She smiled as she uncovered one of her favorite pieces. It was a gnome she had named Saturday Afternoon. Saturday had been posed stretched out next to a tree stump and looked very comfortable. As she looked at the expression on his little carved face, Maggie became firmly convinced that the gnome had always been trying to tell her to take it easy, to relax. She just might be ready to take his unspoken advice.

She carefully placed him on the table and went back to digging around in the box in front of her. All that remained was packing material and a small red water pistol, a relic of happier times before she had married. She set it on the coffee table next to Saturday.

Maggie gathered up the rest of the scattered packing and stuffed it into the empty box, closed the top and tossed the box towards the front door. Two pieces at a time, she carefully put her treasures into the curio cabinet (finally in the proper spot after four tries). Saturday, looking decadently comfortable, appeared to be right at home back in his place in the center of the shelf. Maggie stroked his little pointed hat then closed the glass door. Just like her gnome, she needed to feel at home again.

She tossed a few more of the empties to the front door then set the next box to be sorted out on the coffee table. She dropped a big beige throw pillow on the floor and sat down on it. The letter opener easily slit the clear packing tape. Right on top of the pile of papers and assorted junk drawer items laid that picture. Maggie picked it up, looked at it and said nostalgically, "Rick, you were a good looking man five years ago."

He had been very different from anybody she had ever met before. He just didn't care. He did what he wanted, how he wanted, when he wanted. He was a free spirit right when she needed a free spirit in her life. High school, cheerleading, track team, and honor roll had given her the "right stuff" for college and earlier she had unpacked the trophies to prove it. College had even been structured for her. She had tackled growing up with calm perseverance. He was so different. She had stability, a degree and a career already started. He still rolled from party to party. She planned for the future. He planned for the weekend. She liked his plans better.

The memories hit in a swirl of sweet and sour thoughts. All the parties and the "kidnappings" on Friday afternoons for long weekend road trips blended with all the pointless fighting over things that as Rick said, "Wouldn't matter to the world in an hour."

The fights always lead to the bedroom, or the couch, or the kitchen counter, wherever the fight ended and the mood abruptly changed. At least for the first couple of years this was true. Slowly, there were more fights for the main course and less sex for dessert. Gradually, they spent more time under the same roof and less time together. Finally, they spent more and more time almost avoiding each other.

A couple of months ago, she was sitting at home, alone, when something on the television caught her attention. It was one of those talk shows where the guests make complete fools of themselves for ratings. The television had been on to provide background noise. She sadly realized that this mindless chatter had now become her life. There was nothing left here for her here but static. Rick didn't look surprised when she told him it was over. He actually looked relieved. It didn't take him long to pack. He moved the next day.

Maggie reached to the glass and brass corner table for the tissues. The tears threatened to start all over again. She set the picture face down to the side and stirred the top layer of the box. Faded, yellow newspaper clippings caught her attention. She had gone to high school with Steve and Jean. They had always had an on again off again type relationship. Once high school had ended and the college years began, she and Jean decided that Steve should have been voted most likely to grow up and live in a bad trailer park. Steve could be charming when he had to sweet talk his way back into Jean's good graces, not to mention her bed.

About five years ago, Jean met someone older, more refined. Maggie had gotten to hear about him, but never had the chance to meet him before Steve and Jean both disappeared. A month later, some poor fisherman hauled Steve's body up from the bottom of the river. The faded article in her hand said that Steve must have killed Jean then himself.

The tears wouldn't be denied freedom now. Maggie sobbed quietly for everything that she had lost over the last five years. She had left her job to go with Rick. They moved around a lot. She was married and wanted to settle down, to have something stable. With Rick, she expected the unexpected; instead he seemed to grind to a halt with her. In the five years they had been together, they hadn't bought a single piece of furniture. They had moved five times and he had eight different jobs. Nothing seemed permanent. Just as she passed this thought, a new image flashed in front of her bringing more tears and even more memories. It didn't matter now whether the memories were happy or sad, this was the time that the tears washed away all of the accumulated road grime of the past and cleared the slate. Maggie cried herself to sleep, but not alone. She slept and dreamed with missed friends, forgotten troubles, and imaginary lovers.

Chapter Three

They had been sitting in a secluded corner booth of the restaurant all evening. Brenda had been swimming in the dark, quiet pools of his eyes for the last hour. Dinner had been perfect. He hadn't ordered a huge dinner. Instead, he had a light meal that had allowed for pleasant conversation. The bottle of wine they enjoyed for dessert provided a spectacular end to the meal and the beginning of a fabulous night. Laughter sparkled in his eyes at her funny stories.

He leaned forward when she spoke. She talked about how her work was a dead end job, but at least it was steady. He seemed to hang on every word. The smile on his full, sensitive lips gently urged her to talk about any topic she could find.

"Brenda, do you have anyone special in your life?" His irresistible voice drifted across the table.

"No, not right now." She smiled with her eyes as she answered.

"No one at all. I find that hard to believe. You are such a lovely woman."

She could feel a blush beginning to rise. He made this dinner an event. It was just so nice to be able to talk to a man. "I did have a boyfriend for a while. We even lived together for about a year, but we broke up. I don't think that I have even seen him in almost a year."

"Do you have family here?" He continued to look interested in everything she had to say.

"No, my family is up in Washington. I go back up there for holidays and family stuff." She said, her fork moving slightly in time to her talking. "What about you, Galen? Do you have any family over here?"

"No. My family is scattered around the world," he said. Galen then carefully shifted the conversation back to Brenda. "So how long have you been down here?"

"Oh, I guess about two years now. I have a nice apartment here, so it's comfortable to stay. Besides too much family too close-," she nodded her head knowingly at Galen.

He smiled broadly and said, "I know what you mean."

The bottle would be finished very soon and Galen hadn't made any advance to continue the evening. He turned to the waiter to settle the check. She watched his delicate movements. She frowned as the worst possible thought she could think of hit her. "Oh God, what if he is gay?"

All the evidence was there. He listened to fine music, drank fine wines, dressed immaculately,

over thirty, and had never been married. He had
to be gay.

"Would you care to join me for a walk?" Galen
asked softly, his voice still cultured and romantic.
Brenda kept half expecting him to somehow lose
his accent.

"It's about time you asked," was her thought.
Her answer was, "How sweet of you to ask, I'd love
to." Brenda finished her thought. "Ok, maybe he's
not gay, we still have a night out working here."

He rose first, walked around and held her chair
for her. Galen patiently waited inside in the foyer
while she made the stop by the little girl's room to
"powder her nose". He held the door open for her
as they left. He even made an offer of his hand as
she walked down the three small steps to the
sidewalk. She made absolutely no attempt to give
him back his hand. They walked down the short
path to the lake and walked beside it. As they
walked, he listened intently. No groping, no
patting, no indication that "the move" was on the
way at all.

Somehow, the conversation had turned to the
disappointments in her life then to her fears. She
felt that she could tell him anything. As he
brushed aside a low hanging tree limb, they
discovered a wrought iron park bench at the tree's
base.

"Would you mind if we sit for a minute?" He
asked in a voice like honey, golden and sweet.

"That would be nice." Brenda responded softly.
It would be more than nice. The night air, the half

moon on the water, and no one in sight all enticed her thoughts. He even brushed off her side of the bench first.

Instead of leaning back, dropping his arm over the bench, and draping it over her shoulders, he turned slightly towards so that he could place his hand over hers at her knee. He looked deeply into her eyes. She geared up for the kiss that did not come. Suddenly, she found herself talking again.

"I've had this dream," she paused, " listen to me, all I've done is talk your ear off all evening. It's getting late and you said you have a flight tomorrow."

"My dear, nothing under the night sky could keep me from hearing about your dream. What you think and what you dream are very important to me. I would love to hear about it." Galen responded gazing directly into her eyes.

The sensation of having her thumb gently massaged finally hit. This had to be one of the most erotic sensations she had ever felt. A slight breeze moved the leaves overhead causing the moonlight to flicker. Her words began to tumble out.

"Well, it's a little embarrassing to tell it. You don't really want to hear all this." She shook her head as she talked. Then she looked into his eyes, she felt him waiting. "Ok, but you asked for it. It's kind of a mystery story kind of thing. A black limo just shows up at my place one night. The driver hands me an envelope and opens the door for me. The note says for me to get in the car.

Once in the limo, I'm wearing this red evening gown that is just to die for. I'm driven around for while. Soft music is playing, but the driver is behind that little glass wall and never speaks. We finally get to this big empty looking building and the driver lets me out and hands me another note that says to go inside. I walk in and you can see the full moon through the skylights."

"What happens then?" He asked over the whisper of the leaves.

"I don't remember, I usually wake up about then. So am I crazy or what?" Brenda couldn't believe she had just told him all this.

"No Brenda, I don't think that you are crazy. I think that you are perfect just the way you are." Slowly and very gently, Galen reached to her face. His caress, a cool whisper across her skin that pulled her closer. She could barely breathe as her eyes closed in almost desperate anticipation. At the touch of his lips, she began to understand how women "swooned" in the romance novels with men like this.

Not the usual pounce of most men, the kiss felt like more of a tease. He slowly kissed each lip and then her chin. Her exhale sounded like a bellows to her as a warm blush began to thrill every inch of her skin. He slowly kissed his way down her neck. Each kiss landed softer and more insistent than the last. She exhaled with even greater force as she felt his teeth slide gracefully across her skin.

Galen leaned back and gazed into her eyes deeply and intently. He gently squeezed her hands as the sounds of people walking their direction became apparent. Her eyes glazed lightly as she looked up the walkway at the approaching footsteps. Galen heard the other couple approaching and, unknown to his companion, he could just barely make out the sounds of their pursuer. His eyes narrowed at the sound. This place was no longer safe.

"Shall we go?" Galen asked tenderly.

The words were said and gone before Brenda could nod her head yes. The soft sounds of a predator hidden in the darkness had finally confirmed Galen's suspicions. Recently, he had read about the occasional attacks in this area. They met an ancient profile that Galen knew well. Those reports had been the original reason for his being here. Out in the darkness lay his quarry; the woman was an unexpected pleasure and bonus.

CHAPTER FOUR

Galen walked Brenda to her car, careful to remain unhurried with her. She clung happily to his arm as they strolled past the restaurant. Brenda smiled at the touching romantic nature of the evening. This reminded her of being walked to the front door after a high school date.

They reached her car. She fumbled with her purse while searching for the keys. She felt the awkward moment settle in. She thought feverishly about the possibilities.

"Thank you for the lovely evening, Brenda. I am sorry we have to end our evening so soon, but I will be back in town in a couple of weeks. Would you care to have dinner again?" Galen broke the silence and made the move to end the evening.

"Yes." Brenda blurted out her answer far faster than she had intended. She took a deep breath then said, "Yes, I would love to."

Galen looked at the night sky then looked sadly at Brenda and sighed. She smiled and felt her heart throb. He was such a gentleman. Not only had he not pushed for more tonight he had let her off the same hook. She leaned forward into him. Her eyes closed and her head tilted slightly upwards. His lips met hers in perfect time. He held her lightly at the shoulders and pulled her softly to him. Simultaneously, they both opened their eyes and smiled at each other.

"Good night Brenda. I will call you." He stressed the word "will" heavily.

"Good night, Galen." Brenda smiled and got in her car. As she shut the door, she debated the wisdom of insisting on meeting him at the restaurant instead of allowing him to pick her up. She started the engine and flicked on the lights. Galen still stood there watching her leave. She smiled to him and waved slightly as she pulled away. She sighed. Next time, he would be picking her up and dropping her off. She would pick how the evening would end at the door.

Galen watched her pull away. His eyes shone in the darkness. The evening had gone very well. There was something about her that he liked. She had character and strength. That would just make his plans all the better. He turned and began walking back to his car, careful to look around in a very casual manner. He had the feeling of being watched.

Galen reached his car and got inside. He looked around the area. A few people moved through the parking lot, but they were not what he felt. There was someone or something else out there. In the rear view mirror, the slight motion of a weather beaten van parked on the far side of the lot drew his attention. Even though it looked dark and empty, Galen watched intently as he realized that from the van the entire parking lot could be observed. It rocked slightly again. Someone moved around inside.

Galen rubbed his face in thought. Tonight was turning out far more interestingly than he had anticipated. Galen began to run the sounds and feelings he had at the bench through his mind. People out for a romantic lakeside stroll after dinner being shadowed by someone or something. Galen continued to stroke his chin. Now, he had discovered some kind of surveillance here in the parking lot. Galen decided to wait. Maybe who was the hunter and who was the hunted would become clear.

After a while, the van started and turned on its lights. Galen watched carefully. It began to slowly drive around the perimeter of the lot. Galen decided to follow it and started his car. The van pulled up to the exit, and then turned onto the street. Traffic was light, so Galen hung back as far as he could to remain inconspicuous. The van pulled into the next shopping center along the lakeside. It found a parking spot similar to the first with good visibility. Galen parked at the far end where he could watch the van in his rear view mirror. After several minutes, Galen became fairly certain that the van had become aware of his presence. Obviously, the occupants of the van were searching for someone from the lakeside of the parking lot. This fact continued to hold his attention.

Half an hour passed and nothing had happened. Galen decided to play a hunch and pulled away leaving the van behind. He drove down to the next parking lot with lakeside access. What he had sensed down at the bench must be what the van searched for. Since he felt certain he knew what stalked this area, the presences of someone else hunting raised numerous questions and concerns. Who could possibly be in that van?

Most of the businesses had closed for the night and the parking lot had nearly emptied. Galen decided to leave. As he pulled out onto the street, the van pulled in. Galen smiled tightly. The van didn't act like the police, but it was definitely hunting.

Galen was about to head back to his hotel when familiar looking headlights appeared behind him. From the rear view mirror, he could make out two large men in the van.

"Good evening, gentlemen." Galen said aloud to the image in the mirror. "And what are we hunting for now?"

Galen went under the next traffic light on the yellow. The van followed. Galen smiled as he turned at the next corner. The van followed. Galen smiled again and said, "So it is a merry little chase you wish this evening. Let's see how much you enjoy a very slow chase down the highway."

Galen turned onto the ramp and merged out into the traffic. As soon as the vehicular shuffle settled into lanes, he held his speed to the speed limit much to the annoyance of the drivers now trapped behind him. After a couple of minutes of this, the van pulled away and continued on its way. Galen continued to check the rear view mirror for a few minutes, but the van had truly moved on.

"I must have peaked your curiosity, but I was not your prey tonight." Galen said to the now gone van as he headed back to his hotel. He had confirmed the purpose of his trip and had a new accounting firm to meet tomorrow.

CHAPTER FIVE

Nearly dressed, Maggie put on a little makeup then a couple of eye drops went in to clear up the left over redness. Last night had felt good. It felt good to finally let go of a lot of baggage from the last five years. It felt good to just sit there and be miserable about everything all at one time; no one to have to explain anything to, no one to have to put on appearances with.

She walked out into the living room and looked around. The place looked a little stark, but it was nothing that a few plants and some careful arranging wouldn't fix. Maggie shoved some left over packing into a box then shoved the pile of boxes out onto the patio. She hunted through the townhouse for her shoes and finally found them along with a belt that would be perfect for today.

"There you are. How did you wind up under the couch?" The belt didn't answer, but it did fit snugly. Now dressed for the adult world, her eyes fell on the small, red water pistol sitting on top of the coffee table. A mischievous grin took over her face as she slipped into the kitchen with it. She filled it with water and put the little plug back in it. Maggie smiled childishly as she put the water pistol in her purse. She wondered if Rob would remember the squirt gun fights in the hall they used to have. She knew that water pistols were childish, but she felt like doing something childish today. She had been a grown up for too long.

The old red car with the "Don't Laugh It's Paid For" bumper sticker pulled into its traditional parking spot as if nothing had ever changed. Maggie walked in the side door, stopped, and slipped her shoes off. She quietly continued down the hall. She stopped at the corner and peeped around quickly. There was no one in the hall. She tiptoed down to the first office door on the right and paused. In the best of action movie traditions, she set down the purse and shoes then leaned up against the wall. She held the red water pistol in a proper two-handed grip. One quick look into the room and she saw her target with his back to her.

She steeled herself and counted silently to three. With exaggerated commando style, she flung herself into the doorway and sprayed an empty chair. Water began flying at her from the right hand side of the room. She aimed again and returned fire as she retreated out into the hall. A tall, slender, young man continued the pursuit until they both ran out of ammunition. In unison, they shook their guns, took aim at each other, fired, and got nothing.

"Maggie, I've told you a thousand times, you make too much noise. You couldn't sneak up on a corpse. Your keys jingle, you rub up against the wall and you breath too loud. Oh yeah, always look to the door side of the room, that's where everybody hides."

"Well, I love you too." Maggie replied with as much indignation as possible and remain grinning wildly.

"Thank God, you're back, now this place will have a little life in it." He said as he opened his arms up widely. Maggie fell in for the hug.

"Well, let me look at you. You've finally put on a little weight. You used to feel like hugging a mop handle," she said after few moments.

Rob obediently stepped back and turned around. The light beard and mustache were a nice touch. They took the little boy edge off his face. He had definitely muscled up a little. As he turned, the rear view was still computer programmer flat. Oh well, he was still fun to hassle and start water gun fights with.

"Damn teenagers." Morley muttered to himself as he passed them in the hall. Rob and Maggie both looked sheepishly at each other then burst out laughing.

A small pile of manila folders waited for her on her desk. Maggie sat down, put her purse away in the bottom drawer then flipped on the computer sitting there. As the machine whirred into life she paged through the top folder. Depreciation schedules, pretty simple stuff, the boss seemed to be easing her back into the fold. Maggie leaned back in her chair and smiled. It felt good to be home.

"Earth to Maggie, Earth to Maggie. It's lunch time." Rob's voice crackled over the speaker.

Maggie looked around and finally focused on the wall clock, 12:10. She looked back at the folders. Only one remained and she had just opened it. She folded it shut and set it back in the IN tray. She stacked the other files neatly then set them in the OUT tray. An office intern would take care of the rest. The interns served as elves around the office. They took care of a lot of things, especially when you weren't there to see them.

She punched the sequence of buttons that activated the intercom on the phone and asked, "Rob, where do you want to eat?"

"A couple of us are just running across the street. Wanna go?" Rob responded.

"Sure, just give me a minute." Maggie tapped the intercom button on the phone and the light went out as she slipped her feet back into the shoes under the desk. She always felt that you couldn't properly work at a computer with your shoes on. She fished her purse out of the bottom desk drawer, stood up, and straightened her blouse.

"Oh great, barbecue and a white blouse. This is not a good thing." Her final observation didn't stop her from heading for the door.

Lunch went well. She didn't spill anything on the blouse. The gossip, of course, proved to be even better than the food. She found it amusing that she just so happened to be one of the top office gossip topics. Marriage, leaving, divorce, and returning are all fertile topics for the office wags.

The afternoon passed comfortably as she input and processed the files. At 4:00, Michael came through the office to remind everyone that dinner would be promptly at 6:00, please be there. He left for the airport to pick up the new "member" of the family. At 5:00, Rob started calling on the intercom about the backups. It amused Maggie to watch as people milled about at the front desk for a few minutes then, almost in mass, headed out the door for O'Brian's. Obviously, Rob wasn't the only one who liked the taste of free food.

The restaurant turned out to be one of those trendy places with the double entry way coupled with lots of woodwork and stained glass. Maggie walked in and paused to allow her eyes to adjust to the light. She walked past the hostess, smiled and said, "I already know where all the trouble makers are."

As she rounded the corner to the private room, Rob and Morley waved her over to their table. As she sat down, Rob finished making his point.

"It's easy. It's easier to do everything on the computer. If you don't like the layout or the screen, I can change it for you. With the new systems out now, it takes almost no time to sort data anyway you want to use it"

Maggie grinned as she looked into Morley's face. He still didn't like or trust "calculators on steroids".

"Listen Rob, I don't mean to put down what you do. I mean the computers can print out great reports. They can fill in the forms, and they can even get it right most of the time, but they can't put things in perspective. We're not just "bean counters" anymore. Things have just gotten too complicated for that." Morley's expression softened. "We don't just account for the past. We provide the information that our clients use to predict their futures. Your machines can only spit out what they are told to. What's that garbage saying?"

Rob patiently replied, "GIGO - garbage in garbage out."

"Yeah, that's it. With or without your fancy computers, if you don't ask questions and follow the patterns in the financials you're looking at, then you're putting garbage in and trying to get gospel out." Morley sat back in his chair satisfied he had made his point.

The arrival of the waitress saved Rob from having to make an immediate comeback. They ordered their drinks, waved, and said hello to a couple more arrivals from the office. Maggie overheard two of the female interns speculating on the age, weight, marital status, and wealth of the new client. Maggie smiled and wondered a little herself. After all, she had recently rejoined the ranks of the single. Rob and Morley kept up their debate until Michael appeared at the doorway. An expectant hush filled the room as everyone turned towards the door.

"Everyone, I would like to introduce Mr. Terrance G. Mircalla. Mr. Mircalla, this is everyone," announced Michael with a dramatic sweep of his arm. Greetings murmured around the room in response.

Michael led his guest to the waiting table. As they sat down, conversations resumed. Maggie looked Mr. Mircalla over carefully. It was easy to see how he made a living as an image consultant. His movements resembled those of a performer on stage, carefully careless. His rich and brilliant complexion fit his well-formed features. He wore clothing that represented two month's salary to Maggie and he wore them well. She watched his hands as they moved back and forth in the air in time to his conversation with Michael. The ring caught her attention. The deep purple stone had to be at least five carats in size. The band bore an ornate pattern. This was not the usual tacky, oversized, gold nugget and diamond ring that most men wore. This was more of an heirloom of old money than a show of wealth. He languidly reached up to the corner of his sunglasses and pulled them off. She expected pale eyes like moonlight, what she saw surprised her. His eyes shone fiercely brown, deep like an ancient forest. She realized she was staring when he nodded his head towards her. Embarrassed, she looked quickly back to her own table. Something about him was familiar, hauntingly familiar.

Chapter Six

Something about Mr. Terrance G. Mircalla bothered Maggie all night. He still dwelled on her mind when she poured herself a cup of coffee in the office break room. Taking a quick sip from her almost too full cup, she walked back across the plush carpet to her desk. Maggie sat down and stared at her screen as if it were a crystal ball. She began to tap her pencil on the desk slowly. Whatever it was she tried to remember stayed stubbornly locked away. Maggie shrugged her shoulders, shook her head slightly, and flipped open the file on her desk. She began punching in data on her keyboard.

Several young people walking to the conference room broke Maggie's concentration from her screen. As she looked around, the last couple of stragglers filed past. She looked at her watch. She had been staring at that screen for two hours already, time for a break. From the look of the conference room, it was also time for one of the company's training sessions for the interns and new staff members. These always proved to be interesting because Derek Lawson, the senior partner of the firm and Michael's older brother, always taught these classes. Maggie rolled her head side to side as she stood. She picked up her cold coffee mug and headed for a fresh cup.

On the way back to her desk, she stopped in the doorway to the conference room and smiled as she looked in. The family resemblance between Michael and Derek was immediately apparent. Derek may be a little heavier and have more gray hair than Michael, but he moved around the front of the room with confidence and ease. He walked back and forth in front of his audience gesturing like an auctioneer as he attempted to pull answers from the crowd.

"All right, let's try this again. This time, don't just read me back the numbers. I can read the numbers. Tell me what they mean. Tina, why don't you try?"

Tina began repeating the numbers on the page. Maggie shook her head. Tina wasn't going to give Derek what he wanted. Maggie heard this routine time and time again during her first year. The pained look on Derek's face just so happened to be the same look she used to get when she tried to answer these questions. Tina gave it a good try, but obviously missed the mark.

"Remember the original question here, people. The client wants to know why the sales in this department are running so hot and cold." Derek's hands moved like a high school band teacher's trying to get something that resembled music out of the crowd. "Now, everybody agrees that sales are not what they could be." Derek nodded his head emphatically up and down until the crowd nodded with him. "We've looked at the store hours and we've gone over the allocated dollars per square foot of displayed merchandise. We've even looked at the inventory turns. Has anybody thought to compare the hourly sales recap to the payroll sheets?"

The blank looks and the sudden shuffle of papers gave a clear admission of guilt that they had not. Derek smiled and glanced up at Maggie. He winked to her then looked like he was closing in for the kill. "Has anybody seen the problem yet? Anybody?"

Derek looked over the room like a vulture glaring down five miles of desolate highway. He stopped and focused on Tina due to the puzzled look on her face. "Tina, what do you see?" Derek leaned forward expectantly.

"Well, sir, I, well, it looks like part of the problem is that every time these two employees' schedules overlap, the sales drop off." Tina shrugged and looked up at Derek.

Derek threw his hands into the air as if signaling a touchdown and gloated, "That's it! All they had to do was adjust the schedule to separate those two employees and their sales increased."

At this point Maggie, still smiling and shaking her head slightly, walked back over to her desk.

The stack of unopened files mutely greeted her as she sat down and got to work.

CSEOEOCR

The telephone/fax machine sitting on the huge cherry executive desk rang once and then again before the nearby hand drifted across the desktop to lift the receiver.

"Hello. Speaking." Galen paused as the caller spoke. "You have found me a site to look at. Very good." Galen paused then continued. "No, I am afraid that I will not be in town until that weekend. If I can impose upon you for a favor, just overnight the key to my office and I will go look it over. When I am done, I will leave the key in your drop box."

Galen nodded his head as he listened. He shifted the phone to the other ear as he picked up the black and gold Mont Blanc pen and began to write down the directions.

"Yes, I am looking forward to doing business with you as well. Thank you and I will see you soon." The amethyst stone glinted in the candlelight as he placed the receiver down.

Galen reached behind himself to the matching credenza and opened the center door. He selected a white pages and a yellow page directory from the stack and set them on the desk before him next to his laptop. Time to get to work. He already had Brenda's home phone number. He looked up her address with a reverse lookup. Next, he pulled down a map of her location. Just for cross-reference, he looked up the same information in

46

the white pages - it matched. Her address now complete, he put the white pages and the zip code book away. He could now set everything else in motion.

The first stop in the yellow pages was the section on florist. He scanned the pages carefully. Never order twice in the same year from the same florist if it can be helped and never order from the small shops. They have a way of remembering details. Internet ordering left too much of a paper trail. Dealing direct made tracing a transaction much more difficult.

With that call made, he leaned back in his chair and closed his eyes. He allowed his mind to recall Brenda. Like the computer sitting there at his side, he began to analyze her. He remembered her height, her weight, and how she moved. He recalled everything about her, down to the finest detail with practiced ease, just like he had analyzed a thousand women before her.

Galen tenderly licked his lips and opened his dark brown eyes. He turned the pages to the limousine services and continued his search. There was a time when all of the preparations took weeks and there was always the risk of being remembered. Now, you just pick up the phone and remain faceless. The system was easy. Just don't use the same business too often.

The limousine transaction now completed - it was time for the dress. Galen opened the drawer in front of him and removed the fine leather billfold and gently closed the drawer as he stood up. He placed the billfold in his sports coat's pocket and put on his gold-rimmed sunglasses.

Today, the world had truly become convenient for his pleasure. All he had to do now was drive down to a major department store and look around for the red evening gown "to die for". He would pay in cash and have the store box and wrap it for him. Then he would find a shipping center with a line waiting at the counter. Normally, the first one he came to would do. The hurried person behind the counter would blend his face with the thousand other faces that they would see today. Anything else he needed or wanted could be easily obtained when he was ready.

The smile on his face began to turn as he remembered the end of the evening. The quiet sounds of stalking played over and over in his mind. He had flown back yesterday to meet with the new accounting firm. Today, he would drive back and see if his prey still prowled the lakeside. If the van was still present and wanted to follow him again, he would be more than willing to play another round.

Chapter Seven

Galen arrived at dusk. He parked on the outside edge of the parking lot. He intensely scanned the area. Everything looked normal, so far. People came and went from the restaurant and its neighboring shops. The van was nowhere in sight. He walked across the lot to the path by the lake. Joggers and other people still occupied the pathway and lakeside. He walked down the path to the bench he had found on his previous visit.

Galen sat down and let the darkness advance across the water. The sounds of the night began slowly. People still came and went, but in smaller numbers. Soon, just isolated couples wandered the path under the half moon. His senses tuned for the small sounds of stalking, he allowed his mind to wander. The van had him concerned. If they happened to be the police, then they would just have to come up empty handed. Galen had a much better use for their lakeside attacker than they did. All they would do is lock him up. That would be such a waste. If they weren't the police, then what did they want? Galen didn't like to share his prey. They would need to just stay out of his way.

After a few hours, the long awaited sounds reached his ears. Galen had trouble making out the heartbeat or the breathing, but that was to be expected. All he needed to hear were the slow deliberate movements of a stealthy person approaching. He readied himself.

"Who are you?" Hissed at him from the night.

"My name is Galen. May I ask yours?" He responded, careful not to turn around or make any sudden movements.

"I've heard of you. What do you want here?" The voice asked from behind him.

"That depends on you." Galen answered calmly. He hadn't moved since his visitor had arrived. "How long have you been here?"

The quiet sounds of movement told Galen what he needed to know. The person behind him stood ready to attack at the slightest provocation. Galen began to relax his body and very carefully uncrossed his legs in order to be ready to move quickly.

"This is mine. Go away." The voiced said harshly.

Before Galen could respond the sound of footsteps could be heard on the path. He gritted his teeth. This wouldn't be a good time for interruptions. He had to just sit there and look happy while the couple walked past. The sounds behind him moved away the other direction.

After they had passed, Galen stood up and looked around crossly. It didn't matter. He had come prepared for this. From his pocket, he produced a pair of cloth bottom shoes and what looked like tan colored weight lifter's gloves. He pulled his shoes off and slid them under the bench. Once he had put the gloves on and rolled up his sleeves, he started off down the path.

Galen pondered as he pursued. If the stalker had been staking out the park for the last couple of weeks, how long before he needed to feed? Probably soon. Galen looked up at the sky. The half moon hung in the night sky with few clouds for company. There was even a nice breeze drifting lazily across the water. This was a good night for hunting.

Galen began to pay more attention to the path. He already knew that there would be several paths leading in and out. Following the van had shown those to him. The main path went completely around the lake and was ringed by trees and undergrowth the entire way. The decorative lighting had been installed sporadically providing plenty of dark recesses to hide in. Galen continued walking. The cotton soles of his shoes made almost no noise to his delicate ears. He flexed his hands and forearms instinctively as he walked. On a hunch, Galen turned up an access path to a parking lot. Small animals rustled through the fallen leaves as he passed.

Galen paused and listened for any small sound that would give this man away, nothing. He couldn't tell which way the stalker may have gone. The best thing to do now was to wait for him to show himself. Galen decided to move the hunt to a baited field. He may have to wait a few hours, but it should be worth it.

The poorly lit parking lot still held a few cars after the regular business hours. Who ever designed this area had no idea about security Galen mused to himself. As a matter of fact, edges of the lot actually had no lighting at all. Even though no businesses remained open there were still employees yet to leave. To his trained eye, this looked as good as any place. He settled in behind some bushes with his back to a tree. He didn't want any nasty surprises from behind.

The lights went out in the front of one store as four people stepped outside. One of them turned and locked the door. They all walked out into the parking lot together. They split up when they reached their cars. They stood and talked for a couple of minutes. Galen watched the perimeter intently. Nothing moved.

Finally, they all got in their cars and started them. Galen smiled. They didn't know it, but by leaving together they may have just saved each other's lives. As the last car pulled away a small movement caught his eye. Someone just walked by the front window of the boutique in the center of the building. The owner or manager must still be in the building. This was exactly what Galen was waiting for.

Time passed and the owner of the last car had still not come out. There had been no movement along the bushes so far, but this all felt right to Galen. A glimmer of reflected light gave notice that the door to the boutique had opened. Galen began to move. He slipped through the darkness quickly.

The woman walked briskly to her car. She had parked out in the middle of the lot. She should be able to see anyone who approached her, but Galen knew better. He moved faster around the edge of the lot towards the woman.

She, blissfully, didn't see anything as she got in her car. She turned the key and the engine started right up. She turned on the lights and pulled away. She went safely on her way home.

Galen knew if the stalker was going to move on her it had to be as she unlocked her car door. He had been right. He was almost on top of him when they saw each other. Galen accelerated to a run as he passed the stalker and turned into the trees. He knew pursuit to be the stalker's only option now. The sounds behind him confirmed this.

Galen kept moving. To stop now would mean a confrontation. He was not quite ready for that, yet. The stalker doggedly kept pace. Galen kept dodging around the trees, moving in half circles. He ran in an elaborate obstacle course while he made a pattern out of his path. The stalker began to adjust to the set escape route. It was just a matter of moments before he cut Galen off.

Galen made an educated guess at when he would be attacked and abruptly changed paths. He caught a small tree as he passed and swung back around to face his pursuer. The stalker headed straight at him. Galen continued the swing around the tree and caught the stalker across the chest with his free hand. The stalker grunted from the impact and stumbled across the uneven ground.

"What do you want?" The stalker hissed out loud as he regained his footing.

"I want to know why you were out here night before last?" Galen answered from a few feet away.

"What I do out here is none of your business, Galen." The stalker breathed hard.

"It is my business when you are stalking me. Do you honestly think that I am going to tolerate that?" Galen said with a commanding tone to his voice.

A low sickly laughter filled the air. "You! Tolerate! And just who do you think you are to talk to me like that?"

"I suppose that is what we are going to find out aren't we?" Galen moved to put the tree between them as he spoke.

"Well, Galen, my name is Trevor. If that means anything to you." He smiled brightly in the dim light. Carefully, he stepped back slightly.

It was Galen's turn to laugh softly in the night air. He stood there silently for a moment then he shook his head and said, "So, you crawled out of your sewer when you felt me go by. What am I to be, your first trophy?"

Trevor looked uncomfortable. They stood there, eight feet apart, like two rams eyeing each other. Trevor may have been shorter than Galen, but he had the stockier build. Trevor was unshaven and dirty looking compared to Galen's still crisp appearance.

"We can't just stand here all night, Trevor. What is it going to be?" Galen decided to push this. He knew Trevor didn't want a direct confrontation. That was their usual way. Galen, on the other hand, had no problem with the prospect.

"Why did you come back here tonight?" Trevor looked like he was ready to try talking.

"I wanted to see who had not cleaned their plate and left some fool running loose that would get us all killed." Galen was willing to lecture if Trevor was willing to listen.

"Go away, Galen, this is my territory, my hunting grounds." Trevor began to look nervously around through the trees.

"We have no territories, no hunting grounds. That gets you captured and I know you don't want that. You have already started attracting attention to yourself. That makes you a dangerous liability to me."

The sound of a car pulling past made Galen turn his head to look through the trees. Trevor bolted back into the darkness. Galen spun to give chase, but changed his mind. Trevor knew these woods too well. A long chase through the woods on foot wasn't Galen's style. He would try a different method. He calmly walked the last few yards back to the main path and stepped out onto it. He brushed his shirt and pants off as he walked. Eventually, he came back to the bench where he had taken off his street shoes.

Galen sat down and slipped the cloth shoes off. He bent over and reached back for the others. He looked tired and hadn't even looked around before he had sat down. Galen counted silently to three before he savagely lunged backwards and elbowed the shocked Trevor in the forehead. He knew Trevor would have to try to kill him before he left. He pulled Trevor forward over the back of the bench and slammed his head into the seat. Trevor's arms flung out at the impact. Galen leapt over the back of the bench pulling Trevor with him. Galen's eyes blazed as he hammered his victim in the midsection. Galen pulled Trevor back under the trees behind the bench. He stood him up and brutally punched him in the back over the kidneys. Trevor collapsed to his knees unaware of the cool mist that seemed to be flowing off him towards Galen.

Galen had been right. Someone had been careless and not finished this one properly. Trevor was a threat. If he had been arrested for his attacks, prison wouldn't have been the answer. Galen's eyes blazed fiercely in the darkness. He wouldn't tolerate competition much less being stalked himself. The arrogance of this upstart enraged Galen further. Trevor had the arrogance of actually attempting to attack him. Galen could feel the energy about him rising. The mists drew him into the finish.

Galen stood behind Trevor and ripped his head to the side. The skin of Trevor's neck was clearly exposed. As Galen lowered his head, Trevor's eyes rolled back and closed.

CHAPTER EIGHT

Maggie walked over to her desk with a small cup of water and poured it into the base of the plant. A few new leaves had opened up over the last couple of weeks. It looked a lot healthier now than when it had arrived. She crumpled up the paper cup and threw it away as she sat down. She punched the power button on the computer and leaned back to sip her coffee while the system whirred into life.

"Ms. DeVane, excuse me, but could I ask you a question?"

Maggie turned around in her chair toward the voice and said, "Of course Tina, what is it?" Maggie nodded toward the chair next to her desk and Tina sat down.

"Well, I'm doing the data entry and set up for the Mircalla account and it's a little confusing." Tina confessed.

"What do you mean?" Maggie leaned forward.

"I'm having a hard time telling the difference between what is business and what is personal. I know everybody around here is always talking

58

about looking for patterns and how it all is supposed to tell a story, but this stuff doesn't make any sense. It doesn't help that this file is only for the last twelve months. I've already called his old accounting firm and asked them for the rest of his stuff. They said that they would send us copies of what they have, but it will take a week or so before they can get it to us." Tina explained.

"All right, go get the file and we'll give it a look over together. Okay?" Maggie smiled as she offered.

"Thanks." Tina said with relief as she quickly got to her feet.

While Tina walked away, Maggie typed in her password and began to call up the proper file. She looked up and saw Tina on her way back. Tina had a seat and opened the file to the yellow post-it note with the question mark on it.

Tina began, "I started by looking through the expenses and setting up the chart of accounts. He banks through several different institutions, but that's no problem. I just set each bank account up under assets. Now, right here is where it gets a little weird, he has a lot of credit cards issued by banks all over the world, but we don't have all of the monthly statements or the receipts. I don't want to just lump all of the charges in one place unless I have to."

Maggie flipped from one page to the next, following the path Tina pointed out. Maggie looked up briefly at Tina and was impressed. To see what Tina saw in this paperwork, a person would have to be bright enough to be confused or an expert auditor in money laundering. Something about Mr. Mircalla still bothered Maggie and this paperwork convinced her that he was not what he appeared to be.

"Tina, I tell you what. Let me look this over for a while and I'll even finish the setup for you, if you'll punch in the Winston account for me." Maggie offered with a friendly expression.

Tina nodded her head and stood up. "Okay, but you've got to tell me how you sort all that out when you're done."

"You got a deal." Maggie agreed as she folded up the Winston file and handed it to Tina. Maggie didn't even see Tina leave her desk. She had already become engrossed in the Mircalla file.

Maggie decided to just start over from scratch. She opened a new file for Mircalla Enterprises on the computer and opened the chart of accounts. Two hours later, she looked at her finished product. He had two accounts per bank spread over fifteen banks. One account was always some kind of checking account while the other was an interest bearing account. Two of the banks were in Switzerland and three banks were in the Caribbean. She made a tally sheet on her note pad. Five of the banks were in Europe, two in Great Britain, one in France, one in the Netherlands, and one in Austria. The rest of the banks had been scattered across the United States. All of the bank accounts showed wire transfers every month between them. The truly odd part happened to be the pattern of bill paying. One account appeared to provide nothing but cash advances for two months then deposits were made to bring the account back to a minimum of $100,000 dollars. The account was left alone for a couple of months then the wire transfers began again. Another account would be used to pay all the business expenses for two months then went into the rotation of deposits and transfers.

From what she found in the check registers, there were at least twenty different Visas and MasterCards being used. The simplest thing to do would be to group this dizzying array of money movements into broad asset and liability categories and be done with it.

The intercom and Rob's voice finally broke her concentration. "Hey Maggie, it is lunch time."

She cleared her head and said, "Thanks Rob. I just have a couple of minute's worth of stuff to finish."

"Some of us are going to go get Mexican. How does that sound to you?" Rob asked.

"Umm, that sounds good Rob. I'll just meet everyone there. I'll only be a minute or two." Maggie lied.

"I can wait for you." Rob offered.

"No, you just go on ahead and I will be there shortly."

"Ok, see you in few minutes. Bye." The intercom light went out.

Maggie dove back into the file. By the time people started wandering back in from lunch,

Maggie had managed to enter the last couple of months' expenses. This man had very good taste. He used a lot of cash and traveled frequently. Maggie tapped the end of her pencil on the desk impatiently. What on earth could he be doing? So far, it looked like he had nothing else better to do, but sit around and play some kind of weird monopoly game with real money.

At 5:00, Maggie backed the computer file off onto her jump drive, folded up the file, then put her purse and coat down on top of it. The company frowned on anybody taking files out of the building, but she hadn't finished with this one. She scooped up the entire bundle and headed for her car.

During the drive home, she kept going over the accounts in her head. He was definitely playing some kind of game, but it didn't fit the usual pattern of money laundering. There were no large commercial loans and it looked like all the credit cards had been paid religiously. Why the strange rotation of funds? All of the income appeared to be tied to invoices. There was nothing that didn't have an explanation.

At home, after changing into sweats and a tee shirt, she opened a frozen dinner, and put it in the microwave. She set the electronic timer and walked back into the room now doing double duty as a dining room and an office. Her personal computer sat in the middle of the table. Maggie loaded the jump drive in the slot after she logged in. The microwave dinged that dinner was ready.

Maggie ate while she flipped through screen after screen of the information that she had entered earlier that day. She sorted the files one way then another looking for something that would give her a clue as to what he was doing.

After an hour of staring at the screen, Maggie shook her finger at the screen and said, "I don't know what you're up to yet, but I'll find out." She rubbed her bottom lip thoughtfully as she closed out the software. She shut off the computer and walked into the other room, flopped down on the couch and turned on the TV. She needed a little down time. She would need to be rested for tomorrow's assault on the Mircalla mystery.

At 8:00, Maggie was already at her desk when Morley walked by with the first of many cups of coffee.

"Well, aren't you here early." He jibed.

"This Mircalla account has me bugged, Morley." Maggie answered with all seriousness. "This guy has money flying all over the globe. It looks like he's laundering it, but I can't figure out how. There aren't any loans that are going unpaid that I can find. As a matter of fact, it doesn't look like he has any commercial or private loans at all. There are a lot of credit cards, but good companies issued them. Everything looks traceable, but we don't have the complete records yet."

"Let me get my chair, old knees you know." Morley said as he toddled off to get his chair. Maggie thumbed the pages impatiently until she saw him heading back her way.

For the next hour, Maggie showed him everything she had set up and what she thought it meant. Finally, Morley leaned back and rolled his shoulders. He turned his head side to side to relieve the stiffness of the morning. His cup had become empty and cold.

"Maggie, what are you trying to ask me? Admittedly, this is the most detailed setup on a chart of accounts in the entire history of the firm, but why?" Morley asked looking at the screen.

"Would you believe me if I said I just have a real bad feeling about this one?" Maggie asked almost pleading.

"Look, a bad feeling is one thing, but looking for trouble is something else. Maggie, he is our client and he's paying for all this." Morley explained.

"I know, but if he's up to something, don't you think we ought to catch it before we have to sit here and watch federal investigators do it?" Maggie continued her pitch, "Besides, if he's not up to anything illegal, there's no harm done and he's paying us to take care of everything."

Morley rubbed his eyes and then sighed in defeat. Maggie looked hopefully into his eyes as he turned to the screen again.

"Okay Maggie, what we have here is one of two things and possibly a combination of both. First, this could be money laundering if the invoices are bogus. That will be easy to check by verifying the paid invoices with any recognizable clients or companies that he may have billed. The other thing is," he paused, "this might be is the worst case of hiding money from ex-wives I've ever seen."

"Ex-wives, you got to be kidding. That ah..." Maggie trailed off into silence thinking about her recent divorce.

"Men will do some pretty amazing things to the stuff that they consider their property. They'll hide the remote to the TV. They'll spend thousands of dollars on an old junk car because it will be a "classic" some day." Morley paused for dramatic effect as he made quotation marks in the air with his fingers then continued. "If a man will sneak into the kitchen in the dead of night just to eat the last ice cream bar, just imagine what a man with money will do to keep an ex from getting her hands on "his" (more quotation marks in the air) money. Anyway you want to look at this, this man is making way too many transactions for a one man business." Morley gestured by waving his hand over the file and her keyboard and then finished, "This is a man with something to hide."

CHAPTER NINE

A note had been taped to her door before she arrived home. After she had gone in and set down the small grocery bag, Brenda took the note downstairs to the management office. A long white florist box waited for her as well as three smiling and very jealous female rental agents. Brenda smirked to herself as she went back up the stairs. There were three boyfriends or husbands out there somewhere in real trouble and they had no idea why. Chances were good that they wouldn't even see it coming.

Brenda shut the door behind her and walked over to the table in the dining area of the apartment and gently set the box down. The vase still sat on the counter from the last set of flowers she had received two weeks ago, the day after her first date with Galen. He had sent her a friendship bouquet that time. It had been lovely and it made her feel special.

She filled the bottom of the vase with water and walked back out to the table. Carefully, she pulled the ribbon off and opened the lid. Inside lay one dozen long stem red roses. Brenda smiled broadly as she placed them in the vase and teased them into a lovely arrangement. There was just something about getting flowers, the way they made her feel special. Brenda didn't know why they made her feel so good and right now she didn't care. She had roses and those three downstairs didn't. It may have been catty to think that way, but it added to her enjoyment.

"Well, Mr. Mircalla, you certainly have style." Brenda said out loud to the roses. Before she could continue, she heard a knock at the door.

A muffled male voice said, "Delivery."

Brenda looked through the peephole and saw a young man with a box standing there looking around.

"Just a minute." She said to the door as she glanced at a certain book on the curio shelf near the door. The book obviously met her unspoken approval and she opened the door.

"Please sign here, ma'am." He said as he handed her the clipboard. She signed the little box on the paper and handed the clipboard back.

"Have a nice day." He said over his shoulder as he turned and walked down the stairs.

"Thanks." Brenda said more to the box than to anyone else. Very curiously, she turned the box over and then over again. Roses first and now this had arrived. Brenda felt like a little girl at Christmas. The wrapping on this new present didn't receive the same careful attention the first box had. Brenda crossed the room to the couch as she ripped the paper open. She set the box down on the couch and lifted the lid. She pulled the white tissue to the side to reveal the red silk underneath.

"Oh, my God!" She sighed as she stroked the cool material. She reached in and held the dress up in the air. It was long. It was slinky. It was even the right size by the label. Brenda held the dress up against her as she swirled around. She couldn't believe he took her seriously. She couldn't believe he even listened to her. She felt smitten.

Brenda was no blushing virgin at her first seduction, but this was really just too much. Brenda fell lightly back onto the couch, knocking the box to the floor. She had just met him a month ago, at the bookstore of all places. They went for drinks the next night. He had been very sweet and very attentive. He said he was in town on business and had to leave the next morning, but he would be back in a couple of weeks. All he did that night was hold her hand above the table. He sent a small "thank you" bouquet to her the next day with note asking her out when he came back into town.

Two weeks later when he called she blurted out "Yes" much faster than she had meant to. That night had been incredible. She thought she was going to have to make him call that game show and buy a clue, but he had finally kissed her. What a kiss! None of that usual clumsy grabbing and groping, not that it would have been all that bad, but that wasn't his style and this man had style. Not only did he look good, he dressed well, talked elegantly, and he listened. He didn't just listen he paid attention.

Brenda suddenly sat bolt upright. She jumped up almost panic stricken, torn from her thoughts. Tonight! The limo would be here tonight! Brenda started off in two directions at once and wound up taking three short steps in sort of a circle before she raced down the hallway to the bath. The dress settled over the couch looking as relaxed as a dress can look waiting to be worn for the first time.

At 8:00 exactly, there came the knock at the door. Brenda jumped slightly as the sound interrupted her review of the finished product. The past two hours had been a wild combination of mad dash to get ready, cursing this man, and anticipation. Of course, nothing was where it was supposed to be on the vanity. There just wasn't enough time to make all the decisions. How much makeup? Were these the right shoes? Would this purse match? How dare he make me do this! He had better appreciate this! This kind of evening needed at least two weeks worth of shopping, but somehow, two hours later Brenda felt happy with the results of her efforts.

The door knocked again. Brenda turned to the bed, picked up her purse and turned off the light as she left the bedroom. She expected her date to be on the other side of the door, instead there stood a very large young man in a chauffeur's uniform.

"Good evening, ma'am. This is for you." He said as he handed her a white envelope.

"Thank you, uh, give me just a minute and I'll be right down." Brenda suddenly felt very nervous. She was about to get in a strange car with someone she didn't know. She didn't know where they were going, but she knew who had better be at the end of this ride. Brenda walked to the couch and picked up a smart half-length black jacket. She brushed off a little invisible dust and put it on. She adjusted the purse strap so that it hung just right. On the way past the curio shelf, she picked up the diary book that she had looked at earlier and put it in her purse.

She could see the car as she came down the stairs. It was magnificent. It was so black that it stood out against the night. The driver opened the rear door as soon as he saw her and offered her his hand as she stepped inside. She slid across the seat to the center and looked around. This wasn't the first time she had been in a limousine, but it just had that feel to it, that feeling of being a movie star or someone very rich. The car pulled out onto the street and soft jazz began playing. This was almost too much. Brenda closed her eyes. She leaned back into the plush upholstery and enjoyed the moment.

After a few minutes, Brenda opened her eyes and looked down at the envelope clutched in her hand. Slowly, she opened it and her lips moved slightly with each word.

Tonight is poor payment for the delight of your company, but I shall endeavor to grant you an evening that you shall remember for the rest of your life.

Galen

Brenda rubbed her fingers lightly over the fine linen paper. This evening had all the elements of a late night movie; the good kind where the girl gets her man, and the movie ends with the big kiss scene. She leaned over to the window and stared out into the street through the dark glass. She could see the people in the other cars attempting to see her in the back of the limousine. The fact that they couldn't only added to the effect. Brenda felt like the mysterious lady in a dark mystery and maybe a little like a movie star.

The city swept by the window as the limousine rolled through the night. Brenda saw less traffic as they turned into the office park part of town. Brenda now became filled with anticipation as she felt her destination approach. A couple of more turns and the limo traveled alone on the road. Brenda felt filled with butterflies as the car slowed and pulled to a stop along side an office and showroom building. The driver got out and walked back to her door. She heard the handle click, as the door pulled open. Her heart beat so loudly that she was sure that the driver could hear it.

"Ma'am, this is where I'm supposed to let you out. If you need a return car just call the number on the card and we will send one out for you." She took the offered business card and put it in her purse.

He noticed her hesitation in taking her hand out of the purse. He added, "Don't worry about that ma'am, I've already been taken care of."

She took his offered hand and stepped out onto the pavement.

"Thank you, the limo is beautiful and it was a lovely ride." She said standing there feeling unsure of what to do.

"Don't forget. You just give us a call and we'll send out a car for you. Good night."

Brenda watched the driver walk to the front of the car and get in. He leaned out the window, gave her a little wave, and one last good look before he put the car in gear and pulled away.

She walked to the front of the building. She stopped for a minute and took a deep breath. Brenda straightened up her posture and set her nerve not to absolutely melt in the first five seconds once inside. As she reached for the door, she paused and looked up at the full moon.

Chapter Ten

The reception area stood empty except for a fire extinguisher holding a silent vigil in the corner. Brenda closed the door behind her. The walls had been freshly painted and the thin carpet had been recently laid. Brenda could smell candles. She moved slowly across the room to the hallway that lead back into the building. She clutched her purse tightly in both anticipation and anxiety.

"Galen." She called out softly. No answer. "Galen, are you in here?" She called out a little louder this time.

With still no answer from the darkness, she began to walk down the hallway. She passed empty office doorways as she moved deeper into the building. Just as worry was about to win over excitement, she saw a glow from under the last door. Brenda stopped just in front of it and took what may have been the deepest breath of her life. She slowly exhaled, straightened her jacket, and then turned the doorknob.

As the door swung open, Brenda gasped. Candles had been arranged on two side tables. White sheer curtains blew slightly in the air. They seemed to glow in the tallow light. In between the curtains and the candles lay a white tablecloth that appeared to be floating on air. This apparition had been set with a tray filled with small fruits and cheeses along with a bottle of wine accompanied by two crystal glasses. The faint odor of chocolate drew her attention to a small white ceramic bowl suspended on a brass stand over a small candle in the center of the table.

Brenda stood completely silent and rooted in the doorway trying to take in the scene laid out before her. It was really too much to believe at one time. After remembering to close her mouth, she took a small step into the room.

"My dear, you look absolutely delicious tonight."

The honey dipped words seemed to come out of nowhere and everywhere at once. Brenda barely kept from screaming by covering her mouth with both hands and her purse. He leaned against the wall just to the side of the door.

"Galen! You nearly stopped my heart. My God! You scared me." Her anger melted with the last word as she fell into his arms. They kissed with abandon for what seemed an eternity until Brenda decided to come up for air. Galen tenderly pushed her to arm's length and traveled every inch of her body with his eyes. Everything about her met with his obvious appreciation.

"I hope the dress meets with your approval."

Brenda looked down at the royal red silk material embracing her trembling body. "It's gorgeous. This is all really too much. I..."

Galen interrupted her as he gestured grandly out into the room. "Well, how did I do?"

Brenda slapped his chest in mock anger and kissed him again. This time, she kissed him with insistence. Without words, her tongue told him that he had done very well, so far.

"I can't believe you did this. I mean, I really can't believe you did this. How did you do this?" Brenda stammered after they ended the kiss.

Galen gently took her hand and turned her towards the room and answered, "You tell me about your week first, then I will tell you how I did all this and why."

Brenda, still shaking her head and protesting her disbelief, allowed herself to be shown to the waiting table. Galen guided her to her chair and pulled it out for her. He helped her out of her jacket and even hung it up on a small brass coat rack that until now she hadn't noticed.

Brenda looked around the room again. She smiled broadly. During the day with the lights on, this may not have looked like much, just some curtains, a few chairs scattered about, and a couple of tables here and there. However, at night, with a full moon outside and candles the only light inside, the scene became pure romantic magic. She didn't know where to begin.

"Galen, you're spoiling me. What are you going to do for an encore?" Brenda smirked slightly.

"Have you ever had fresh chocolate dipped strawberries before?" Galen asked instead of answering her question. He smiled broadly.

The whole scene had begun to overwhelm her again. She simply nodded her head "no". Galen selected a small yet full strawberry and lifted it by the cap. Gingerly, he swirled it around in the white bowl. The aroma of warm chocolate filled the air. Once he appeared satisfied with his effort, he lifted the warm succulent treat. A thin line of the vibrant red still showed between the green of the cap and the darkness of the molten chocolate. He held the strawberry steady over the bowl until the excess languidly dripped back in. The air, already spiced by the candles, now swam with the sultry sweet scent of the confection currently being held hostage by his long, sensitive fingers.

Slowly, he leaned towards her and lifted his gift to her waiting lips. Brenda found herself utterly enthralled in the whole ceremony. She waited until it nearly reached her mouth before her lips moved. He paused just in front of her and waited. She could feel her eyes become glassy as she parted her lips to the proper width. Her lips longingly touched the warm, soft chocolate. She only took in about half of its length before her eyes locked with his. She exerted just enough pressure to pierce the skin with her teeth. Just enough to taste the sweet mingle with the tart. Her eyes narrowed into a determined look as she bit through. With his gaze still firmly locked, she swallowed her trophy.

Galen lifted the remaining berry to his lips, never wavering in his intense gaze into Brenda's eyes. The sides of his nostrils flared slightly as he regarded his prize as one would a fine wine. Slowly, he parted his lips and began to lick small amounts of chocolate from the skin. Brenda's attention became enthralled in watching the dexterous tip of his tongue at its work. Feeling that he had completely captured her attention, he slowly enticed the berry into his mouth and gradually covered the berry and the chocolate with his lips. Seeing Brenda leaning forward, her breath held, he hesitated for a moment then completed the act. With a barely seen movement, the severed cap fell away. When he swung his hand loosely away, Brenda remembered to exhale. Her breath came in short choppy waves as she could feel a blush rise slowly up her cheeks.

Brenda gathered her strength as well as her composure for just a moment, then, she reached for a strawberry of her own. She selected the closest one to her and gently yet firmly grasped the moist leafy greenery. She slowly pushed the fruit into the yielding chocolate and began to move it from side to side. As she lifted it out, the aroma became stronger in the room. Brenda stared intently at the tip of the strawberry as the dark viscous fluid swirled into the last droplet to trail off into the bowl. She turned the berry up to prevent any further escape. A fine line of chocolate fell across her fingertips. Her gaze rose to meet his. She waited until she was confident that she had his attention trapped before she offered her gift.

Galen's gaze began at the confection and leisurely wandered up her bare arm to her shoulder. From there, it unashamedly traveled across her breasts, which had begun to rise and fall with a heavy rhythm. Finally, he allowed himself to be impaled on those eyes. As she raised the fruit to his lips, he leaned in to meet her. He was not bashful. He took the entire berry between his lips and softly took her hand with his.

Effortlessly, the strawberry surrendered to his teeth. It was not until she saw him chew twice and swallow that she realized that all she held was the cap. Before she could move her hand, she felt a coolness across the back of her fingers as Galen set about the task of cleaning the spilled chocolate from her hand. The sensation caused her spine to tingle and her eyes began to close as a soft moan escaped her lips.

The gentle kisses and tongue caresses continued up the back of her hand and around to the wrist. The full lip contact at her wrist released a massive surge of warmth that raced down her spine. Her breath drew in as if she had tried to inhale all the air in the room at once. The next kiss on the forearm resulted in her exhaling in one short burst after another. She began to stroke his hair with her free hand. Brenda had no idea that her arm could be so erotic. No one had ever taken this much time or care to cater to her. The kiss on the soft skin of the biceps interrupted her train of thought.

Only dimly aware of standing up for a moment, Brenda found herself reclining into a very padded chair. By the angle and padding, this piece of furniture had been very carefully chosen for a very specific purpose. As he leaned in and kissed her lightly behind the ear, it was a purpose that she was more than ready for. It seemed like years and yet like mere seconds that undivided attention was paid to her neck. Her hands rubbed his shoulders in encouragement. Slowly, the gentle kisses worked their way down to her breasts. The material of her dress seemed to fade into air at his touch. Each of the now exposed breasts garnered equal attention. Slowly, the entire surface was kissed and then the nipples teased lightly. Galen ran his tongue lightly around the ring, inhaling slightly. The sensation rapidly grew in pleasure to nearly the point of pain. Just when she felt she would have to stop him just so she could catch her breath, he would take the entire tip like the strawberry and allow her to exhale.

Gradually, he moved down to her abdomen. The muscles responded to his touch by quivering and jumping. A sultry thrust into the navel caused Brenda to rise up and clutch his shoulders in gratification. Her knees abruptly separated and gripped his ribs as the warm pressure continued. As the first wave passed, she collapsed back and rubbed her hands deeply into his hair resisting the temptation to pull with all her might. Even though she was ready to finish this, she was not in control. An irresistible force swept her along and all she could do was enjoy the ride.

She thought her heart would stop when she felt the first touch of his lips at her upper thigh. His hands kept her breasts from feeling deprived. They also kept her firmly in place. It was plain that he was not done yet. Brenda's eyes felt heavy and slow. The room looked hazy and dim in the candlelight. She could feel his tender and insistent attentions below. Beyond control, she allowed the next wave to overcome her. All she could do was close her eyes and moan.

As she opened her eyes, she felt the pressure against the inside of her thighs. Then a new sensation swept over her. It was like nothing she had ever experienced before. She felt the room spinning and growing darker. The candles grew dimmer. She felt as if the world were draining away. She closed her eyes and let her hands fall away from his head. As her legs relaxed, she could feel the pressure increase against that thigh. She barely felt the fringe of a tablecloth tickle her fingers. Her last thought was that she was cold, so she pulled the tablecloth over to use as a blanket, then the universe faded away.

Chapter Eleven

The day had gone exactly as planned. The rental van had been ready. All of the ordered items were ready to be picked up. The setup had been simple and the end result proved to be impressive even to his jaded eye. Tonight had become something special. This woman possessed spirit and strength. She might even be strong enough to survive rebirth. Galen toyed with the idea for a moment, then gave himself over to the thought that this feeding would satisfy him more than other feedings had in a very long time. That fool, Trevor, had been the main course for this month, but that was not a leisurely feeding for pleasure. That had been for survival.

Generally, most of his food was weak of spirit, easy to snare, but not much of a prize. Rarely, he happened upon one made vulnerable by circumstance, but not weakened or corrupted. Some of his choices had no doubt improved the stock by removing them from the breeding population.

He sensed her arrival as a blend of anticipation and anxiety. Fear was not present and that pleased him. He had grown tired of the taste of fear. It had become too easy to achieve. Tonight, he would attempt to complete a feeding on sexual arousal alone. When he saw her, his dark instincts nearly overcame him. It took everything he had to maintain control. She had no illusions as to why she was here. That inflamed his need for her. She had responded magnificently to the entire evening. Once he had begun to feed, he had become intoxicated with her.

He felt the pressure on the sides of his head lessen as the strength in her thighs drained into him. Her hands fell away from him as the feeding neared completion. He heard the contents of the table fall to the floor, but paid no attention. He hadn't been this enraptured in feeding in many years. He didn't see the chocolate that had served his purpose so well spill out onto the floor. Nor did he see the small, white votive candle that had kept the chocolate in a molten state roll slowly across the thin office carpet to the sheer curtains.

Galen heard the slight whoosh of the curtains bursting into flame. He felt the heat. Enraged at the interruption of his meal, he lifted his head away from the wound he had opened painlessly in her upper thigh. Blood darkened his teeth and lips as he snarled at the flames. At that moment, Galen cursed all things modern such as the fire alarm that had begun sounding. The second set of curtains went up in flames, nearly encircling the couple.

Galen crouched back away from the flames and looked for an opening to escape their embrace. His head whipped back and forth looking wildly around the room. He gazed at Brenda through fear stricken eyes. She still reclined in the padded chair, the silk dress pooled around her like a bloody shadow. The tablecloth had been pulled across her upper torso like a child's security blanket. Her legs had closed as if in modesty. The expression on her face reflected her current pleasant dream.

The wail of the alarm tore Galen's attention away from the still breathing Brenda. The fire would have to finish the job of releasing her from this world. People would be coming. There was no time to finish this evening properly. Galen stepped to the end of the chair, cringing at the rising flames. The candles and their stands now added to the blaze. He looked down at Brenda. She deserved better than to burn to death. He would be merciful. He reached out to her.

"Is anybody in here?!" The shout from the other side of the door stopped Galen's hands from reaching Brenda's neck. Galen made his decision. Just as he moved, the door burst open.

"Damn!" The security guard shouted in reaction to the bizarre scene of fire, tables, and the chair in the center. "Tim, get in here! I need some help! There's somebody in here."

"I'm coming!" A second uniformed man shouted as he entered the room.

Brenda's lovely semi-nude body kept the men from seeing a figure fling itself from the corner out the door, away from the searing flames. The men kicked the standing curtain rods away and rushed to the chair. The first one to her pulled the dress around her like a towel.

"I got her feet. You get her arms and let's get the hell out of here!" The first man yelled to the other.

"All right, I got her. Let's go!" The other man answered. Together, they carried her down the hall to the front room. They set her down gently on the new carpet.

"Tim, grab the fire extinguisher and put that mess out. I'm gonna see if she's okay." The first man instructed the other.

"Ok, Mac." Tim answered quickly. He gave her and his partner one last quick look then moved. He grabbed the fire extinguisher from the corner of the room and headed down the hall. As he entered the back room, he started spraying the white foam over the flames. As one set of flames smothered, he kicked over the remains and moved deeper in. After a couple of minutes, the fire was out. The carpet had been badly burnt and the ceiling tiles would need to be replaced, but the building itself escaped damaged. The fire seemed to be mostly some kind of nylon curtain and a hell of a lot of candles. Tim stopped moving the debris around with his foot and looked back toward the doorway. He hoped the woman they found was all right. They needed to turn off that damned fire alarm.

Mac pulled off his windbreaker and balled it up into a pillow then placed it under her head.

"Hey lady, you okay? Come on, talk to me!" Mac pulled her dress back together in the front. He held her hand and looked worriedly into her closed eyes. He wondered what was she doing in there and with whom. She obviously had been with company in there. Maybe she was the one in the limo he saw drive through a little while ago.

"Come on, lady, wake up and tell me you're gonna be all right." Mac tried again. With this last request, Brenda's eyes fluttered for a moment and she moved her body slightly. "That's it, lady. You hang in there and we're gonna get you some help." Mac sounded hopeful.

Galen's lips tightened in frustration as he watched from outside. She had been rescued and now it looked like she would survive. The process his kind referred to reverently as rebirth would begin shortly. He couldn't leave her here. She had to be taken and destroyed. While he silently cursed tonight's events, he saw her hand move. In spite of himself, Galen smiled slightly. He had always been a good judge of possible candidates. He knew this woman had strength.

"That's right, you're gonna be all right. Come on, don't you dare give up on me now, lady." Mac kept up the encouragement and his hopes. She seemed to be getting paler, but she moved more. Mac hoped she had not gone into shock or overdosed on drugs. These days, who could tell what was going on?

Mac heard a sound at the door and barely got his head around in time to see a blur of movement. Galen had him before he could react or cry out. He grabbed Mac by the throat and pulled him in close. Mac tried to resist, but he found himself swept along. Galen covered his victim's mouth and nose to stop any sound from escaping. The blood to Mac's brain was completely cut off by Galen's grip. Mac kicked out with his feet and pulled at the hand on his throat, but to no avail. The room began to spin as Mac passed out. His last sight was the woman lying helplessly on the floor.

Galen stood over the fallen guard and looked at Brenda. He tried to make up his mind. The sounds from the back room had now become quiet. The other guard must have put out the fire. Galen frowned. Her purse was still back there. Nothing could remain as evidence that she had ever existed.

"The fire's out. Is everybody okay?" Tim shouted up the hall, no answer. Tim looked up the dark hallway and saw two figures on the ground.

"Hey, Mac, you okay?" He called up the hall. "What the hell are you doing?" Still no answer came from the front.

Suddenly, very concerned, Tim quickly walked back up the hallway. The impact at the doorway was so intense that his body flung into a horizontal position while airborne. Tim's inert form struck the ground heavily, like a bag of mulch thrown from a truck.

Galen opened the door on the right in the hallway and picked up a large duffel bag and walked with purpose to the back room. He had a lot to do and he knew he didn't have long to get it done.

Two minutes later, the full duffel bag was loaded in the van. Galen pulled to the front door and put the running van into park while he stepped in and looked at Brenda still lying on the floor. Her eyes had opened now, but unfocused. Her breathing had grown stronger.

"Well, it looks like I am going to keep you after all, my dear. Although, I do not envy you your next few days, don't worry you will live. Not like you think, but you will live." Galen tenderly lifted her from the floor and backed out the door with her in his arms. He wrapped a mover's blanket around her in the back of the van and shut the door. As he climbed into the driver's seat, he could hear the approaching sirens. He smiled as the van pulled away from the building. He would have loved to have heard the two men he left unconscious in the building explain what they had seen.

CHAPTER TWELVE

"You put the coffee on yet?"

"Good morning to you too." Maggie answered sarcastically as she turned in her chair to face the familiar voice. "And yes, the coffee is ready."

"Did I ever tell you that you were always my favorite around here?" Morley answered in his best fatherly tone.

"Yeah, every time I get here before you and make the coffee. While you're in there, be a love and get me a refill." Maggie handed him her empty coffee cup.

"It would be my pleasure. Are you still picking at that Mircalla file?" Morley squinted to see the screen from over her shoulder.

"Of course." Maggie turned back to the screen and tapped on the glass. "There is still something about this man that is bugging me. He may be just trying to stay ahead of ex-wives and girlfriends like you said, but I still think he's up to something more."

"Well, he may be and if he is we'll find out." Morley looked in the empty cup in his hand then walked off towards the break room. Maggie barely had time to arrange the next stack of papers to be entered before she saw Morley heading back with a pair of coffee cups. He tried not to spill her cup while he attempted to sip from his. By some well-practiced minor miracle, he made it to her desk without spilling anything.

"Here you go." He said as he carefully handed her the full cup. "I have a few suggestions," he paused to sip his coffee. "Check this guy's invoices and investment income. If you find something fishy, we'll know he's moving money illegally. If you can, check his travel itinerary from the credit card charges against the invoices to see if they match up. If all of that checks out, look at the interest rates and exchange rates between currencies. He might be playing some kind of system to maximize the short-term returns on his accounts. If all of that works out let me know and we'll both start doing whatever he's doing. We'll make money the old fashioned way. We let someone else do the work for us." Morley winked and smiled as he turned to walk to his own desk.

Maggie, smiling turned her attention back to the screen. It was time to finish out the chart of accounts and get down to some real work. She looked into the white banker's box piled nearly full sitting on the floor and sighed. It looked like a long day ahead at the keyboard.

Maggie leaned back after a couple of very intense hours staring at that screen. She twisted her head from side to side then rolled it back and forth. Next, she rubbed her wrists and looked at the screen again. Assets, liabilities, income and expenses filled the chart of accounts on her computer. She scrolled through the "look up" screen watching intently. Account after account scrolled by. She had never seen anyone live like this man did. She had certainly handled more money than this before, but never anything this spread out before. It was as if he wanted to create as much busy work as possible. There was so much paperwork that anyone would be tempted to dump everything into general categories and call it a day. Maggie didn't know why she was being so hard on this one case; there was just something about Mr. Mircalla that didn't sit right with her.

Tina checked in a couple of times during the morning to see if there was anything she could do. Maggie suspected that Rob had asked Tina to make sure that she took a break from the computer every couple of hours. Maggie had brought her lunch in with her so that she wouldn't have to leave the office. While the intern made her rounds, Maggie ate her sandwich, and sorted out the next stack of papers by date.

The chart of accounts was now set up to Maggie's satisfaction. She would be able to track this guy's every transaction. Maybe Morley was right and Mr. Mircalla was just hiding his money or practicing some weird system of investing. It didn't matter to Maggie. There was just something about this client that held her attention and she was determined to figure out what.

Two hours later and she had made good progress on punching in his actual transactions. From the beginning, there seemed to be a pattern to what he was doing. Maggie split the receipts with Tina, giving her careful instructions as to how she wanted this file entered. Tina, filled with intrigue, got straight to work. Between the two of them, they finished the box by late afternoon. They settled down at Maggie's desk to review what they had done.

Maggie punched several buttons on the keyboard watching the screen carefully. She sat back in her chair and looked at Tina, who also watched with obvious anticipation. She picked up the stack of deposits and invoices then handed them to Tina.

"Okay, I'm printing out the journal on his transportation. What I need you to do is to match up as many of the travel receipts to the invoices as possible. We need to see where this guy is going and if he gets paid for going there. I'm going to check out these transfers and see if he's making any money moving money."

"No problem." Tina replied as she stood up with her stack of papers. "I'll see you in a little while."

Maggie nodded as she watched Tina leave. With an eager look, she began chasing money transfers around the world. She printed individual account recaps. As the sheet of paper emerged from the humming laser printer, she took the first transfer and began tracing its movements.

Just before five, Rob made his announcement over the intercom that it was time to make the daily backups. Maggie leaned back in her chair. Frustrated, she complied with the request to close down the system after she sent a copy of her work to the printer. She roughly punched out her code on the keyboard and exhaled heavily. Hours of looking at this stuff and nothing outstanding could be found. There was a lot of movement, but all the transfers added up. There were no mysterious overages or shortages to follow. Basically, it looked like this guy just liked to have a checking account close to wherever he happened to be and he liked to be a lot of different places.

Maggie picked up the impressive looking stack of paper that just finished printing. Almost dejectedly, she began to page through. Transfer after transfer, bank after bank, some of the transfers made good business sense, but other transfers didn't make him any money. It was as if he had made the transfer out of habit instead of an attempt to make money. Mr. Mircalla made money; there could be no doubt about that. However, why all the money movement if there were no clear motive? Maggie kept pondering these thoughts until she sensed someone standing at her desk. She looked up to see Tina standing there looking considerably less perky than this morning.

"I started matching up the invoices and deposits like you said and they match up fine. Being an image consultant pays pretty well and he has an impressive client list. Mostly foreign corporate types who want to look like old money and still be able to sell to Americans." Tina said tiredly.

Maggie looked at the stack of paper on her desk and sighed, "So, what you are telling me is that this account is going to be a lot of busy work, but nothing truly out of the ordinary."

"I don't know if this is anything but there's a strange pattern of cash withdrawals that matches up to his travels." Tina explained as she scratched her head.

"What kind of pattern?"

"I knew you were going to ask me that, so I asked Mr. Morley to take a look at it. He's got the paperwork in the conference room spread out all over the table. Come on, I'll show you." Tina motioned for Maggie to follow her. Maggie stood up with a tired determination and followed the younger woman to the conference room. As she entered, Morley was still intently playing some kind of bizarre game of solitaire with the papers on the table. He looked up as the women entered and gestured to them to sit down.

He turned to them and announced, "This is the way to make a living, work two weeks then go on vacation for two weeks."

Maggie shook her head and asked, "Morley, what are you talking about?"

He ignored her question and asked her a question instead. "Did you find anything in the transfers?" Seeing her shake her head no he continued, "I didn't think so. Our Mr. Mircalla seems to be a creature of habit. He travels out of town about once a week for a couple of days. The first week is usually business and the trip generates an invoice. The next trip is usually around the weekend and always to a different city than the first trip. The third trip of the month usually generates an invoice and the fourth trip is to a new city."

Maggie and Tina watched Morley's presentation. When he paused, they looked at each other then back to him. Morley pointed to different stacks of papers in time with his explanation.

He continued excitedly. "Now, it takes a couple of months to figure out the cash advances. Once a month, he always returns to a city he has recently visited. On that day, he makes his cash advance. Now, this is the unusual part, once he makes the trip with the cash advance, he doesn't go back there again. At least, not that I can tell from the records that we have here. He may be strange, but he's not breaking any laws that I know of."

"So, why all the accounts, transfers and credit cards," Tina asked.

"Some people just enjoy playing these kind of games just because they can. Although, judging by the places he goes and what he charges his clients, I think I'm going to get me a thousand dollar suit, work up that European-continental accent of his, get me a big fancy ring, and go into business." Morley concluded by folding his arms across his chest and looking indignant.

The word "ring" moved through Maggie's mind looking for a point of reference. After a few futile moments, she suddenly made a very frightening connection to Mr. Mircalla's ring in her memory. The thought didn't make any sense to her yet, but the chance that it might seemed to pull her out of her fatigue. She began thinking very quickly.

"Tina, aren't we receiving his records from a firm in London?" Maggie clinched her hands as she spoke.

"Yes, yes we are. They're sending us the rest of this year. What are you thinking?" Tina asked looking at Maggie's hands.

"Good, I need you to get them on the phone and tell them that we need the last five year's records and we need them as soon as possible. Tell them we have an audit coming up." Maggie had a very determined look on her face now.

"Five years? Maggie, what do you have in mind? A full audit? That's not in his agreement with us." Morley said looking perplexed. "We shouldn't even be spending this much time or manpower on this account."

"I know, but I need to see the travel records. As much as he travels, I want to see how stable he is. He's moving around way too much, even for the idle rich." Her tone left no room for debate.

Maggie didn't tell Tina or Morley that the travel and the ring seemed to fit into a memory from her past. A memory in the form of an old newspaper clipping she had just folded up and put away in a box at home. That ring was the reason she felt something funny was going on.

"It could take a week or longer for the information to arrive." Tina responded.

"What are you thinking, Maggie?" Morley asked looking into her eyes.

"I'll tell you as soon as I can check something in that paperwork." Maggie knew that once she saw those travel receipts, she would be able answer their questions as well as her own.

Chapter Thirteen

She had the sensation of moving or being rocked like a baby. She had been fading in and out of that feeling for some time. She could open her eyes, but she couldn't understand anything she saw. Nothing seemed to focus in her mind, so she just went back to sleep.

As Galen drove, he could hear her moving around a little in the back. It wasn't too late to change his mind. He could stop anytime along the way and dispose of her, but if her body were found now, well, this evening had gone badly enough already. To be honest, this whole month had gone strangely. First, he had to put down Trevor, then that van with its unknown occupants appeared, now this debacle. There was so much to do, so many things that he would have to get for her. It had been several decades since he had a consort. If nothing else, it would be interesting for a while. He took the ramp from the interstate back into town. He and his new guest would be home in a few minutes.

Brenda finally realized that the van had stopped. No matter how hard she tried, her extremities just wouldn't respond. She couldn't feel her arms or legs, just a pervasive numbness. All she could do was lie there and stare at the roof of the van. She tried to talk, but her tongue had become so swollen that speech proved impossible. She tried desperately to remember if there had been an accident. The whole night seemed blurry to her memory. That had to be it. She must have been in some kind of car wreck. Strangely, that thought felt almost comforting. At least it gave her something to hold onto as her eyelids began to slide shut by themselves again. Her parting thought was to hope someone found the wreck soon.

Galen began to unload the van as soon as the automatic garage door closed. He set the duffel bag down in the back corner and picked up a couple of large bags of dry earth from the neat stack against the wall. He opened the door to the house and disappeared inside. Galen carried the bags through the house and down the stairs to the basement. As he entered the basement, a red light bulb began to glow, activated by the motion sensor mounted against the ceiling. Galen set down the bags and looked around the room for a moment. He walked over to the large wooden shipping crates stacked against the wall.

There were six of them, each four foot long, three foot wide, and three foot tall. They would serve his purpose. He pulled the top two from the stack and set them on the floor side by side. He carefully set the lids back on top of the stack. He knocked the end off the first crate with a sudden strike of his hand against the inside wall. The second crate received the same treatment. Galen placed the ends on top of the lids then pushed the boxes together to form one long box. He walked over to a small gray metal toolbox, opened it, and removed a hammer along with a few nails. He took the ends and nailed them over the seams of the new box. Finally, he opened the bags of soil and poured them into the box. After spreading the fine soil evenly throughout the box, Galen stepped back and looked satisfied with his work. Brenda's new home looked ready for her.

Brenda's eyes slid open as she was being lifted out of the van. She tried to smile at the thought that someone had found the wreck. Next, her eyebrows furrowed up as she tried to remember what wreck. It felt like someone was carrying her, but she couldn't lift her head to see who it was. She tried to look around, but she had trouble focusing. Brenda grew even more confused because what she could see didn't look like a hospital. It looked like somebody's house.

"Why would somebody take me to their house?" Brenda thought as her eyes began to roll upwards again.

Galen gently carried her down the stairs into the basement. The red light appeared upon command as they entered. Very carefully, he set her down on the floor next to the box in the center of the room.

With a graceful motion, he sat down next to her and lifted her head into his lap. For several minutes, he simply sat there slowly stroking her hair, lost in reminiscence. As he closed his eyes, the memories of far too many years began to fly by. Galen recalled past consorts, compatriots, and vanquished foes with equal relish. He recalled more impassioned times. The centuries stored in his memory flew past. He could still remember the village of his human birth and he vividly remembered the sensations of his rebirth. He opened his eyes and allowed them to slowly wander over every inch of the body in his lap. He could feel the first tremors of the muscles under her soft skin. He knew that rebirth had already begun.

Tenderly, Galen reached for the one button and the belt that held the silk about her body. He slid her free of her clothing and held her nude body to him. Her warmth had just begun to fade. He rose easily to his feet with her draped across his arms. Like a caring mother placing her child in a cradle, Galen placed Brenda on the soil. Dropping to one knee, he looked intently at her. He searched for the signs that she would survive rebirth now that it had begun. The skin on her face had begun to look tight and swollen. Her nipples stood hard and erect. Her entire body had begun to pale. He reached in and lifted her hand. The arm moved freely, without the slightest resistance. The skin still felt soft and supple. After careful inspection, he almost lovingly set the hand back down.

"Well, Brenda my dear, it looks like you will be with me for a while. If you will excuse me, it appears that I will have arrangements to make and I have a little shopping of a sort to do." Galen turned to leave, but was drawn back to the box by a slight sound. He looked back in and he saw her eyes flicker then open slightly. They shone blood red and very painful looking.

Brenda thought she heard someone talking to her so she began the long climb back up to where she could open her eyes. She tried twice and failed. With a final act of desperation, she wrenched her eyes open as best she could. The insides of her eyelids had to be made of sandpaper as they scoured their way across the eyes. There was nothing to see but red. Something must have happened to her eyes in that wreck. Now, if she could just remember what wreck. A sensation of heat followed by a chill swept across her body causing her to moan.

The movement of her tongue caused her pain that so intense as to become an exquisite sensation. She would have moved, but nothing seemed to be attached. She couldn't even sense her skin. She thought this must be how one of those isolation chambers must feel. She wondered what kind of drugs she had been given. She saw something move. It wouldn't come into focus, but it started to talk to her.

"You are far stronger than I thought, trying to wake up at a time like this. I do not envy you the next few days. That strange feeling that you have now is your body becoming something new. We call it rebirth because you are emerging into a brand new world. As we speak, I suppose that modern medicine would say that you have an uncontrolled viral infection that is invading every cell in your body. It will keep what it needs and it will eliminate what it does not. Picture, if you will, an antelope becoming a cheetah. That is what is happening to you. If you survive rebirth, you will be a wholly new person. Be strong, Brenda, and I will see you soon."

The talking red thing disappeared from view and for just a moment she could hear his footsteps, his breathing, and even his heartbeat. He faded from hearing range. Brenda lay there alone and confused until a single scarlet tear trailed from the corner of her eye, staining her pale cheek with its passage.

Chapter Fourteen

Galen needed to return the rental van first thing that morning. He carefully cleaned all the vinyl and plastic surfaces with a spray cleaner and a rag. He paid extra attention to all the small areas underneath the dashboard, doors, and the seats. These were areas that he or Brenda may have left fingerprints and never known it. Once satisfied with the wipe cloth, he set up the portable steam cleaner. The upholstery may have looked clean, but the wastewater was black with dirt and potential evidence. He would return this van far cleaner than when he rented it. Hopefully, the next customer would lay down a new layer of dirt, fingerprints, and other traces of themselves, making Galen's trail cold if not impossible to follow.

He had parked his car in the lot across from the car rental agency. This bit of careful planning prevented anyone from driving him home and possibly remembering the way or the passenger. He had just walked back in the house when the phone rang.

"Hello. May I help you?" Galen answered the phone. "Good morning, Mary, and how are you doing today?" He really hadn't anticipated her to call this quickly. "No, I was not planning on coming out until this weekend. Is there something wrong?" Galen smiled at the real estate agent's distress. "The building was damaged last night. How terrible."

The phone call from her about the building was almost humorous. Galen sympathized with her. He told her that it was a shame that the building was unable to be rented for now. It was shocking that kids would have broken in and started a fire. No, he would not be interested in another property. Yes, next time he needed a facility, he would call her first. The woman seemed to want to prattle on for hours. He had grown tired and needed to rest. Galen finally succeeded in getting off the phone with her. Just as he had leaned back in his chair, the London accounting firm called. They needed his approval for something about releasing information to the American firm. He crossly told them to send them whatever had been requested, just don't call again today. He had just changed American firms and now it looked like he would have to change the overseas firm as well. Tired and annoyed now, he left the office and walked through the house to his bedroom.

He undressed, slid under the covers, and exhaled deeply as he lay there in thought. He could feel the pressure beginning to mount. This country had become too curious and computerized. The thought of the strange van still disturbed him. Trevor's existence had been a warning. Someone out there had gotten sloppy. Always clean your plate was the morbid motto. He closed his eyes as he thought of Brenda and everything letting her live would entail. He yawned and gave up thinking. It felt good to be in his own bed.

Galen woke up at dusk feeling better. Then again, he always felt better after feeding. He didn't have time to dwell over all that fate had twisted so strangely. There were a lot of arrangements to make. Galen dressed casually for the evening. The light-blue oxford-cloth button-down worn with the tan slacks meant he would look nice, but not be memorable.

He parked the black, year-old Acura at the edge of the town square, next to the park, away from the streetlights. What he was shopping for tonight could be found locally. He began walking down the sidewalk into the darkness of the park. Only the faint scratch of his fine leather soles on the concrete gave warning of his approach. The faint sounds did not matter. Tonight didn't require stealth.

He found himself breathing deeply in the night air, actually enjoying the walk, and the search. Without the pressure of feeding, this was simple; find what you're looking for and leave. Tonight reminded him of simpler times before the world had modernized with cars, computers, and cell phones taking over daily life. No planning and evidence to destroy or hide, you simply set out to find your prey. When you found it, you claimed it.

He snapped himself out of his nostalgic flight of fancy and back to the business at hand. His walk had taken him away from the lights, back to where people wanted to be veiled by the darkness. The night was alive with signals and sounds for anyone who took the time to be aware. The muffled sounds from the other side of a row of bushes happened to be a young couple heavily entwined around each other. Galen smiled, from the sounds of things, they knew very little of what they were doing.

As he continued down the path, the all too familiar sound of being stalked reached his ears. When you prowl the night, you run into others hunting under the cover of darkness. Of course, he had done nothing to avoid nocturnal predators. He walked alone down an isolated path in an unlit part of the park. Galen didn't possess a massive stature and his clothing clearly indicated he would have money and credit cards in his possession. Galen sighed. When you looked like prey, you couldn't blame the opportunists for wanting to take a bite.

Galen began judging his pursuer, young, wearing athletic shoes. The faint rub of denim from his legs confirmed blue jeans. His breath sounded tense, but not heavy, so he was not a novice at this type of activity.

Galen wondered what method of attack would be used. The path was coming to a split. To turn right would be to head back towards the lights and apparent safety. To turn left would mean to go deeper into the park and the darkness. Galen turned left.

He could hear the young man stop pacing him and move across to intercept him at the next turn. Galen heard the young man's breath steady and the leaves rustle slightly as he positioned his feet. Galen continued walking as if oblivious to the world.

⋘⋙

As tonight's victim stepped on the colored path square that served him as a trigger, the young man hurled himself forward from behind the bushes. It only took him two steps to reach his target. He swung the mini-bat in his right hand with all his might at the man's head. Instead of the usual heavy thud, which was supposed to happen now, his wrist suddenly felt as if it were caught in a vice.

He still moved forward with momentum when he saw the man turn back towards him. The impact of the man's other arm across his throat slammed into him so hard that he felt his feet ripped from the ground. Next, he felt his body driven like a spike into the concrete of the path. At the moment of impact, he felt the bones in his wrist separate. The pain from his wrist allowed him to feel the living hell his hips, spine and neck had suddenly become. All he could do was moan and throw the other hand up in front of him as a shield. The man dropped the other arm carelessly.

⋘⋙

Galen almost tenderly took the offered hand and with a swift gesture rendered it the same treatment as the first. Before the young man could cry out, Galen dropped to his knees and grabbed the young man's throat, stopping all sound. The gentle pressure on the proper spots on the throat delivered blissful unconsciousness to the young man in a matter of seconds. Galen released his hold and rose elegantly to his feet. His eyes flashing and his nostrils flared, Galen felt alive.

He looked down at the body lying there like a broken toy and smugly said, "You are very fortunate this evening. I am giving you the chance to make something else of your short life since you will no longer be able to pursue this line of work."

Galen smoothly looked around the area. Without haste, he listened for any movement that may give away any witnesses. Only the normal night sounds of the park bore witness to the dark events. Satisfied, Galen grabbed the would-be assailant by his collar and easily dragged him around the edge of the shrubbery away from the path. Galen let go of the collar and unceremoniously dumped the man to the ground. Galen walked back out to the path, the broken man on the ground already forgotten.

After a few more minutes of walking, Galen finally neared his destination. This side of the park had a thick line of trees that acted as a buffer between the park, the traffic, and the commerce of the city on the other side. Due to an unused partially covered drainage culvert, this area attracted the homeless, usually transient men. These were the people that most people hoped disappeared.

Galen stepped off the pavement and onto a well-used footpath under the looming trees. Galen could hear movement ahead. Cautiously, like a hunter not wanting to spook the prey, he moved ahead.

This first one turned out to be too old and diseased for Galen's purpose. The next one he found was a woman, tattered and road weary. Galen could smell wasted blood on her. She had probably been fighting. She looked up at him as he walked by. She raised her hand to her hair and patted it down in a futile attempt to look more presentable. Galen studied her face as he passed. She had been a nice looking woman not too long ago. Her scent revealed her need, a chemical beast that had destroyed everything else in her life. It always amazed Galen at the ability of some humans to continue living long after the will to live had vanished. Something unspoken passed between them as their eyes met for just a moment. She looked away and huddled back into her corner. She didn't want what he had to offer, yet.

Galen found a young man sitting and rocking. He mumbled something to himself as he rocked back and forth on the ground in perfect rhythm to his unintelligible words. He was a very large man, far too large for what Galen needed, but something about him held Galen's attention. Galen couldn't sense alcohol or drugs on this man. He was mentally ill and, therefore, condemned to this life. Perhaps, he had chosen this over his other options. Galen stood there and watched as the man continued to rock back and forth and mumble. Galen turned and walked away as the man petted a small dog that was not there.

After passing by a few more of the choices lining the path, he saw what appeared to be a possibility. The man slept up under the edge of the culvert. Galen stopped and listened to his breathing. He snored slightly. His breathing flowed easily, not labored. The scent was unwashed, but not heavy with alcohol or drug abuse. Galen leaned down and took his hand gently. The pulse felt sound. The flesh seemed to be in fair shape, not too weak, or too strong for his purpose. He, obviously, had been on the road for a while, but not so long that he had begun to truly deteriorate. Yes, this one would clean up nicely. Galen patted the hand until the man stirred.

"Don't be alarmed, I have a proposition for you. Are you interested?"

"Wha?" Came the groggy response. The man rubbed his hands across his face trying to wake up. As his eyes focused, he saw a nicely dressed man staring back at him.

"What did you say?" He asked slowly.

"I said that I have a proposition for you. Are you interested?" Galen asked again, trying to look friendly. His potential choice seemed to still have most of his mental faculties.

"What church are you from?" The man asked as he sat up.

"Church? Oh, no. This has nothing to do with coming to church." Galen explained. He was amused at the question.

The man rubbed his eyes again and looked at the person in front of him. He didn't look like the church type. He also looked too clean to be the kinky sex type, but he had a funny accent. Then again, these days, who can tell? "What do ya want then?"

"A friend of mine is doing a thesis on American society. I agreed to help her find different kinds of people to interview. We would like to interview you and possibly a few of the people you know out here." Galen sounded convincing.

"What's in it for me?" The man asked as he looked suspiciously at Galen.

"Room and board for a couple of weeks and possibly a little money at the end of it." Galen explained.

"Then what?" He pressed.

"Then nothing. You go your way and we go ours." Galen's look changed from friendly to annoyed. "We are not trying to save anyone. We will feed you and house you for a couple of weeks and pay you for your time, but if you are too busy right now, I am sure that I can find someone else down here looking for food and a clean bed." Galen stood up abruptly and turned to walk away. The interruption came just as expected.

"Wait a minute! I didn't say no. Look man, I just woke up." He explained. This was happening to quickly for him to think it through, but what was wrong with a meal and a bed?

Galen smiled then returned to his best friendly face and turned to the man. "Well, come on then. Dinner is on me."

Chapter Fifteen

Brenda began to hear a powerful sound. It didn't make any sense to her. As she concentrated on the sound, it became a great pounding. It came from nowhere and everywhere. It was more felt than heard. The sound grew louder, like an immense sledgehammer landing on unbreakable stone. The sound was either getting louder or closer. She couldn't tell which. The moment she decided that the sound was getting louder, it stopped. Brenda was confused. What happened? She took a deep breath and the pain began. Her heart caught in a vice and wouldn't beat. She could feel the soft tissue around her heart begin to tear under the strain. To scream would have been at least some kind of release, but the sound caught in her throat and refused to escape. Her hands wouldn't respond. All she could do was lie there motionless, helpless. Only her face reflected the internal turmoil. The pressure continued to build. The weight on her heart continued to grow.

Every time Brenda thought that it could get no worse, the sensations increased. She knew that her heart had been crushed and now her lungs felt as if they had been set on fire. She knew that she couldn't possibly be alive. No one with a crushed heart lived, but if she had died, wouldn't the pain have stopped?

There was a final tear and then nothing for a moment. Brenda could feel her heart begin to sluggishly beat. It didn't feel strong; instead, it felt soft and blubbery. Every beat continued to be sick and lethargic. Brenda began to panic. Why didn't somebody help her? Where was she?

Brenda tried to open her eyes, but she couldn't tell if they were open or not. She saw only darkness. She couldn't feel anything except the horribly degenerated beat of her heart and the fire now burning in her lungs. She could find no other sensations. She tried desperately to feel anything else and found nothing. Brenda finally tried to escape by flinging her mind out into the blackness.

At first, Brenda was relieved at the lack of feeling. The soul rending pain had finally ceased. She enjoyed the sensation of floating out into the warm blackness. She could hear nothing. She could do nothing. Someone must have given her a painkiller, but she couldn't remember why she was in so much pain. Thinking was not going well for her either. Thoughts simply wouldn't hold together. No matter how hard she tried, memories just wouldn't come into focus. Floating around not connected to anything rapidly began to lose its novelty.

Brenda found herself becoming angry. That seemed to work, very well. She became enraged at being helpless. Images began to come into focus. As they floated up to her, she struck out in boundless rage. In her mind, the images did not bend or brake; they were torn, ripped to shreds. The more she destroyed, the more images appeared. The more that appeared, the more enraged she became.

The images became more and more bizarre. At first, they were simple faces or images of places. Now, the images began to twist into nightmare shapes. The peaceful face of a long dead relative now laughed in bizarre mockery. She attacked it. Brenda lashed out again and again until it had been shredded. She walked naked into a room full of people. They began laughing and pointing at her. She blushed, and then cried. Still, they laughed at her. Her rage flung her at the images. They screamed at her brutality and ran through the blackness. The more they screamed, the more brutal her attacks became. Brenda became enraged at having to chase them down and kill them. She tore them to horrifying, quivering little pieces. Her rage seemed to know no boundaries.

All about her lay the gore of her rage. The blackness itself became the target. She tore at it. She clawed her way across the carnage. She began to see a statue of a woman through the haze. Brenda forced her way to it. It wouldn't come to her the way all the other images had. She reached out to touch the unreal shape. She felt the pull of being drawn back in.

Gradually, far off in the distance, she began to hear the pounding again, slower than before, but stronger. The grip of iron that previously held her heart had faded. The pounding settled into a steady rhythm. Brenda found this calming to her rage. It didn't end the rage. It merely allowed her to contain it. The fire in her lungs still burned brighter than ever.

Her heart seemed to be slowly growing stronger, but now Brenda had difficulties breathing. The air felt forced into her lungs. The pain grew to an intense burning sensation deep inside her. The lining of her lungs peeled away from the walls, exposing the new tissue beneath. She could tell by the area now burning that this was going to go on for hours. She felt the strike of the first wave of wracking coughs. As she coughed, the affected muscles beneath her taunt skin seized and cramped, twisting her body into surrealistic shapes. This proved too much for Brenda to bear. She simply gave up trying to live. She flung herself back out into the blackness again.

This time, she hid from the pain. Brenda pulled the darkness around her like a security blanket and watched the images fly by. Everything that she ever remembered now displayed itself as a mockery. Everything she had ever thought now twisted into new directions. The good in her life seemed to be all gone.   All that remained was the searing pain and the rhythmic pounding in the distance.

Chapter Sixteen

Galen brought his prize back to the house. David Langston was his name. He had introduced himself during the ride. They didn't talk much in the car past the introductions. David dozed in and out as they drove. He stayed awake once he realized that they had left the city and headed out into the suburbs. The houses kept getting larger and further apart as they drove. Finally, they turned off the main road down a side street. David didn't see a street sign and the area lacked streetlights. At the end of the street, they turned down a nearly hidden driveway. The exterior of the house impressed David. He was going to spend a couple of weeks here - in a nice house telling rich people how bad it was out on the streets. David smiled wondering how long he was going to be able to stretch this out.

As the automatic garage door closed, Galen turned to David and said, "Follow me inside and I will show you to your room."

"Yeah, sure, whatever you say." David tried not to look too excited about the words your room. It had been quite a while since he had heard anything like that. He was actually having a little trouble believing his luck. He was still homeless. He still had all of the same problems. For right now, he didn't care.

His host led him into the house. It turned out just as big as he thought it would be. There was, however, much less furniture than he expected. The house seemed to have just enough to get by. Probably just renting David decided. The bare walls echoed their footsteps as they walked down the hall to the last door on the left. Galen opened the door and stepped aside like a bellboy for David to enter the room first. The room was sparsely furnished like the rest of the house. It reminded David of a nice hotel room with no frills, except for a television and DVD.

"You will find the bath through that door over there. There should be soap, shampoo, a razor, and anything else you might need already in there. There are clean clothes in the closet. Feel free to wear anything that fits. Are you hungry?" Galen inquired looking concerned

David only half listened as he looked around. "What? Um, yeah, I guess I'm a little hungry."

"Well, you go ahead, and get cleaned up and I will go see what we have to eat."

As Galen turned to leave the room, David looked directly at him and said, "Hey, look man, uh, I really want to thank you, this is all really great."

"Don't worry about it. I'm just doing a friend a favor, just like you are going to. Now go bathe, and I'll call you for dinner." Galen still looked concerned. In truth, he was most concerned that David bathed before dinner.

David watched his host leave and close the door. He didn't hear it lock. He almost expected to. David began looking around the room again. He walked over to the closet door and opened it. The closet was well stocked with men's clothing. David saw his reflection in the mirror mounted on the inside of the door. His clothes hung layered and filthy. His hair had matted to his head and his beard was uneven and ratty looking. The bags under his eyes didn't look all that bad compared with the eyes themselves. They were bloodshot and runny. Over all, he looked like hell's leftovers.

Leaving the closet door open, David walked over to the bathroom. He gasped as he flicked on the lights. The room was clean and tidy. The recessed, whirlpool bathtub seized his attention. He walked over and sat on the edge of the tub. He set the temperature on the water and put in the stopper. As the tub began to fill, he stood up and began to peel the material from his body. Piece by piece, he dropped the road weary clothing into the hamper and, finally, slid his grimy body into the warm water.

He looked around briefly until he found the controls for the tub. He punched the "on" button and was rewarded with effervescent, swirling water. David settled back and melted into a look of complete satisfaction.

Galen stood thoughtfully in the kitchen. He wondered where to start. After several minutes had passed, he heard the water being run in the tub. David would be in the tub quite some time; at least Galen hoped he would. He finally decided that this decision didn't require this much thought. He opened the drawer next to the refrigerator and pulled out a dark metal plate and ran hot water over it. Once it had warmed, he dried it and set it on the counter. Next, he opened the freezer section of the refrigerator and pulled out two plastic-wrapped, filet mignon from his favorite stockyard in Chicago. He set them on the metal plate. They should be defrosted in a few minutes.

A hand full of almonds went into a pot of simmering water. He cut up a small onion and put it into a covered bowl. He lovingly wiped down the excellent quality knife before he returned it to the wooden block holder with the other assorted knives necessary to have a well-ordered kitchen. Galen took down another pot and put two cups of water on to simmer. From the cabinet to the side, he took out a box of rice mix, opened it, fished out the spice packet and poured the rest of the contents into the water. Sliding his thumbnail along the edge of the packet, he slit it open easily and poured the contents in with the rice. A couple of quick selections from the spice rack and he looked satisfied. While the modern trend in prepackaged food made life convenient, he regarded the foodstuffs as a good place to start in a pinch, but extra care was required if you actually intended to eat it.

A couple of more trips to the freezer and a little attention paid to everything already out had dinner nearly ready. Galen thought while the modern world had its drawbacks, the quality and quantity of food available today was simply incredible. Having to rely on the seasons for eating choices ended only a few, short decades ago. Today, fresh blueberries from New Zealand sat on the grocer's shelf in February, while live lobster swam in tanks year round.

Galen checked the heat settings on the dinner then turned and walked across the dining area to the other side of the house and down the stairs. He used his key at the door, then descended the basement stairs. The motion detector turned on the red light at his approach. He stopped at the bottom of the stairs and gazed at the grotesque form sitting statue-like in the center of the box.

Her hair, matted and full of earth, stuck out at odd angles. Small, dark blood spatters covered her body and the inside of the box. Her back had arched impossibly backwards with her face up toward the ceiling. Her arms were outstretched and the fingers had locked into claws in the air. The muscle definition had become more pronounced. Galen moved towards her and walked slowly around the box. He could barely detect any breathing. She must have been fighting the metamorphosis. The expression etched on her face was one of rage and pain.

Galen reached out slowly and just barely touched her shoulder. She felt like skin over brass. She still had the paths of her bloody tears showing on her face and down her neck. Under the red light, this all looked like a macabre tattoo. Galen closed his eyes as he remembered his time and wondered if he looked like this.

After a moment, Galen turned and walked back to the stairs. As he climbed, he didn't look back. The path had been set and it was too late to change it at this point. Galen had survived this long by being careful and trusting fate every once in a while.

Once in the kitchen, he checked to make sure everything had proceeded smoothly. Each item met with his satisfaction. He opened a bottle of tawny port wine to let it breathe. He went ahead and poured himself a glass and took a sip. It was a rich almost fruit wood flavor. It was an unusual choice. Galen didn't normally drink Australian wines, but this one seemed to match his mood. He sat down in the dining room and stared into the darkness.

David punched the "off" button to the tub and just sat still as the last of the fine bubbles died away. He looked at his clean fingernails and his wrinkled fingers. He had been in the tub a long time. As a matter of fact, he thought he might have fallen asleep for a little bit. He stood up and rubbed down with what may be the finest feeling towel that he had ever felt. Maybe the towel wasn't that good, but it felt great to be clean again. David wrapped the towel around his waist and walked over to the vanity. The mirror showed progress, but there was still work to be done.

He trimmed away the longer facial hair with the small scissors on the counter then lathered his face. The new razor exposed clean, fresh skin with each passage. David lifted water up in his hands to his face and rinsed the rest of the lather off. As he removed the towel from his face, the mirror showed him someone he hadn't seen in a very long time. He took the scissors carefully to his mustache. Next, he began to drag the brush through the tangle of hair. It was longer than he thought, long enough to pull back into a ponytail. David opened the medicine cabinet and there on the bottom shelf he found the little rubber bands for hair. He never could remember what they were called.

David stared at the almost forgotten face in the mirror. How long had it been since he had been clean? A growling sound from his stomach reminded him that his host had mentioned dinner. He walked back out into the bedroom and immediately enjoyed the carpet under his bare feet. This was a sensation that most people never noticed, but he had gone without it for so long it became a major event. As he stood in front of the closet and looked for something suitable, he opened one of the drawers in front of him. It was full of underwear. David had nearly forgotten how good a pair of new, clean, cotton underwear could feel. While it was truly material happiness, he had begun to think that he was never going to be clean again and now tonight.

After pushing the hangers back and forth for a minute, David decided on a white full shirt with a mandarin collar and a pair of dark blue slacks. He tucked the shirt in and looked at himself in the mirror. He held out his arms and turned slightly from side to side watching his reflection. David smiled as he decided that he looked good in white and blue. A pair of black slip-ons with white, cloth soles that looked about the right size sat in the bottom of the closet. David picked them up and walked to the bed. He sat down and slid them on. They were a little big, but they would do.

The aroma of roasting meat crept slowly into the room. David's stomach immediately reminded him that it had been a while since the last meal. He stood up and walked to the door. With his hand on the knob, he looked back across the room with disbelief. A couple of hours ago, he had been asleep in a park. He had nothing to do and nowhere to go. Now, he was late for dinner.

Galen heard the tub shut down and begin draining. He went back to the kitchen to begin the final arrangements. He turned on the grill in the center of the stove. While the grill warmed up, he checked the rice. It looked and smelled good. On the sideboard, the rolls had risen. They went onto a baking sheet and into the oven.

The almonds were drained, then the onions and a packet of freshly frozen French-style green beans were added with a little water. He selected a small knife from the block and carefully opened the plastic around the meats. He put the rich, red meats on a plate as he threw away the assorted packaging on the counter. Once the counter had been cleared, he reached into the spice cabinet above the stove and selected an antique, silver, pepper grinder. He liberally ground on the red and black specks. A quick pass of his hand over the grill confirmed that it stood ready and waiting. As the fillets touched the hot metal grill, a loud hiss and a great cloud of steam rose into the air. Mentally, Galen timed everything and opened a far cabinet and drawer. From these he gathered everything he needed to set the dining table.

As he returned to the kitchen, he could hear the soft footsteps in the hallway. "How do you like your steak?" Galen asked David as he approached.

"My what?" David's stuttered his reply.

"How do you like your steak; rare, medium or well?" Galen asked again with clarification.

"Ah, medium, I guess." David answered in surprise.

"If you would like to have a seat, go on into the dining room." Galen gestured towards the room.

"Is there anything that I can do?" David asked as he stood in the doorway staring at the food.

"No. I think I have everything under control in here. Go ahead and make yourself comfortable."

Galen replied as he stirred the green beans on the stove.

"Uh, okay," was all David could manage as he crossed the room. The unbelievable turn of events this evening had him off balance. He walked over to the table and stared. It had been set with a white tablecloth and real silverware. The bottle of wine sat open and there was half a glass on the table. David sat down and poured himself the other glass. He leaned back and took a sip. There was no bitter bite to this wine. He took a deep breath and gently shook his head. The smell of bread cooking became almost tangible as he heard the oven door close. He took a longer sip of his wine. This time, he truly enjoyed it.

"Are you ready to eat?" Galen inquired from the kitchen.

"Yeah. Sure am." Before David could add anything else Galen turned the corner carrying two plates. He served the plates to the table with practiced ease. David looked down at his plate. Fresh rolls, a steak with bacon on it, green beans with almonds, and that fancy rice stuff like they have in restaurants. He just sat there unsure of what to do. There were too many forks. He suddenly felt very uncomfortable. Galen smiled from across the table as he looked at David's face.

"Relax, table manners do not matter here. Go ahead try something." Galen urged.

"Sorry, I'm a little nervous. This is all great. The shower, the clothes, and now the grub. I can't pay for this." David stammered.

"I told you, I'm doing this as a favor for a friend. As a matter of fact, I believe she will be here by tomorrow night. Now go ahead and try something, so you can tell me what a fabulous cook I am." Galen glanced from David to his plate grinning.

At that, David visibly relaxed, picked up a knife and fork then launched into the plate. David didn't even look up for several minutes. Galen ate lightly while watching David closely. He still had the basics of manners and had cleaned up well. By this time tomorrow night, his body should have started to clean itself out. Galen was pleased with his choice.

Galen leaned across the table and poured David another glass of wine without asking permission. David smiled a thanks to his host as he spooned in another mouthful. They didn't talk much during dinner except for the occasional thanks from David and the demure denials by Galen.

They finished their plates almost simultaneously. Galen had served David nearly twice as much as himself. He knew the man would be famished. Galen had kept his glass filled and watched David's eyes grow heavier. By the end of the meal, David looked full and very complacent. At Galen's insistence, they finished the bottle. He needed to wash all the grime from this man's system and he really didn't feel like a lot of small talk after dinner. He wanted to retire before dawn. Galen knew that he would have a long day ahead of him tomorrow as it would be Brenda's third day and, by the looks of things, she would be up early.

At first, Galen was half tempted to give David rules like don't roam around the house on his own, but it didn't matter. It was Galen's experience that people like David would sleep most of the next day. Their bodies would be trying desperately to make up for all the neglect of their lives. Besides, everything he didn't need to see was already under lock and key.

David felt sleep overcoming him even before they finished that bottle. He said his goodnights and wandered back to his room. David lay down on the bed; safe, clean, warm, and full. He drifted off to sleep smiling.

Chapter Seventeen

After David had gone to bed, Galen cleaned the dishes by hand then placed them in the dishwasher. Old habits are hard to break, especially after a few hundred years. He pulled several plastic bags of fresh fruit from the refrigerator. He set them on the counter and rummaged through a cabinet until he found a curious three-part bowl. Ice went in the bottom part while a nice selection of grapes, strawberries, and plums filled the middle section. Once the lid had been replaced, the ensemble turned into a self-cooling serving bowl.

Galen took the bowl and walked down the hall to David's room. He eased the door open and stepped inside. Without a sound, Galen walked to the dresser and set down the bowl. He could hear the gentle snoring from the bed. David lie there fully clothed with the top cover pulled over him. Galen crossed the room to the bathroom. Without any lights, he walked directly to the hamper. From a panel on the outside of the hamper, he took out a new bag then removed the full bag from inside.

After installing the fresh bag, he took the old one and gave David one last glance before closing the door.

Galen took the bag of clothing down to the garage and put it in the garbage can. He picked up the duffel bag from the previous night and carried it back up to the study. He would unpack it later when he had more time. He walked down to his bedroom and sat on the edge of the bed after locking his door. He yawned widely and then undressed. As he slid under the covers, he looked forward to tomorrow. It would be a busy day.

Galen didn't wake until after two in the afternoon. He sat up and looked good-naturedly at the clock. He had over slept, but he felt good so the clock was forgiven. He stretched and arched his back until he heard and felt the popping of his spine. He rolled his head from side to side and yawned. His lips curled back to expose his very white teeth. His shower, shave, and dressing were leisurely pursued. A simple collarless gauze shirt in caramel with black baggy pull-on pants insured he would be comfortable for the rest of the day.

A quick check on David revealed that he still slept soundly. That meant Galen still had plenty of time. His next stop was the mailbox. It had been a couple of days since he had picked up his mail and the box had been stuffed full. He carried the pile of envelopes back to his study. He quickly sorted the mail with most of it going into the wastebasket. He didn't see anything that required his immediate attention so he moved on to the duffel bag. After a cursory search, the only thing he removed was Brenda's purse. He set it on the desk, the rest of the bag he took with him to the kitchen. The candleholders and the rest of the glassware went directly into the dishwasher. The small white bowl now covered in hardened chocolate went directly in. He added in the soap, closed the door, and started the cycle. Amazing things, dishwashers, they eliminate fingerprints and evidence of all types. The high temperatures and harsh alkaline detergents destroyed most organic trace materials and even did a fair job of sterilization. No trace of the other night would remain at the end of the cycle. As an added bonus, the equipment even cleaned the dishes.

He laid out his dinner for this evening. A few boxes, a few cans, and a couple of items from the freezer placed in the sink made up his choices. He pulled a couple of bottles of wine from the rack. He felt the need for an exceptional wine to go with tonight's menu.

A feeling in the back of his neck told him it was time. He checked on David again. He still slept. Galen went to the basement. He locked the door behind himself then descended the stairs. The red light was already on. Someone or something had already tripped its signal. Galen stood on the stairs listening intently. All he could hear was the easy rhythm of breathing coming from the box in the center of the room. He walked slowly forward and peered in.

Brenda, no longer trapped as some twisted piece of modern art, lay on her back with her eyes closed. The spatters of blood had extended their range to everywhere in the box. The soil beneath and around her had been kicked around and scattered, but it had done its job of soaking up the excess fluids eliminated from her body.

A strong odor of decay had permeated the room. Galen got a small brown folding chair from a box leaned against the far wall and had a seat. It wouldn't be long now.

He watched the rise and fall of her breasts over the next hour as they slowly swelled to over three times their normal size. Her face quickly bloated to unrecognizable proportions. It appeared as if her entire body had gained about two hundred pounds in the past hour. Small rivulets of blood began to run from the base of her finger and toenails. A faint popping sound from her right foot and the nail on the big toe tore loose under the pressure. The rest of the nails on that foot quickly followed. The left foot and then the hands all soon began the same process. Small rips began at her nipples in the skin. Tiny drops of clear liquid ran from the seams. Her nipples, a light pink an hour ago, had turned a dark brown. They became so distended that they looked as if they were going to explode. The lacerations continued spreading down her breasts and stomach. After a few minutes, her entire body ripped from head to toe. The skin peeled away in sheets, clinging to her body in wet clumps.

As quickly as the swelling had begun, it began to recede. In the areas not shielded by the sheets of dead epidermis, a new, clean, skin showed through. It was without blemish as it shrank back down towards the body that waited for its snug embrace. As the hands and feet receded, new nails began to show. They were longer and stronger than before.

Galen had quietly witnessed the events in the box unfold. As he watched, the new skin continued to shrink. The strange process had nearly completed. Her muscle tone had improved dramatically. Her body now bore all the hallmarks of a long distance runner. As the new skin dried, the curve of her hips returned, as did the fullness of her breasts. She stirred slightly as if sleeping.

Brenda was having the strangest dream. The images that had haunted and tormented her seemed to be gone. It was night and she was running. She ran forever and didn't tire. She ran effortlessly. She felt nothing underneath her feet, but she could feel the wind in her face as her hair whipped behind her. She ran until she reached a great field. Surrounded by nothing, but picturesque wide-open space, she kept running for the sheer joy of it. She felt no effort on her part as the earth passed beneath her.

She leapt into the air and hung there with no sensation of falling. She perceived that her body had weight, but still she didn't fall. She continued to move faster and faster back into the darkness. Her speed kept increasing until she passed the sensation of movement. She felt oddly relaxed.

Now, she floated along enjoying herself until she smelled smoke.

"Fire!" She screamed as she sat straight up flinging dirt and wet skin everywhere. She sat there unsteady for a moment then collapsed backwards into the box. Galen went over to her body. He reached in and began gently rubbing her down with handfuls of the earth. Once he had removed as much of the dead skin as possible, he moved to the head of the box. He firmly stood her up and held her still. Dirt rained from her in small clumps. He turned her to face him. He bent down and lifted her up on his shoulder. Once he had her up, he turned and headed for the stairs. He would have to clean up the mess in this room tomorrow.

The stairs groaned lightly under the increased weight of his footsteps. At the top of the stairs, Galen paused listening intently for any sound of David. He heard nothing. Quickly, he walked to his bedroom and shut the door.

Galen carefully placed the nude woman into his bathtub. He turned on the tap and checked the temperature with his hand. Once satisfied with the water, he stood and removed his own shirt exposing the same type of lean muscles as the body in the tub. He tossed the shirt into the hamper, then turned back to her and the tub. He pressed the "on" button and the bubbles began to swirl the dirty water around her body. Galen took a bath sponge and tenderly washed her down. He took great care not to scratch or damage the new skin.

After a few minutes and a filter change for the tub, the water began to clear. Her new body glistened in the wetness as he stood her up and wrapped a towel around her. He leaned her across his shoulder as he released the drain. As the water level dropped, he eased her back down into the tub. Galen patted and dried her with great care as he admired her new shape, lean, muscular, yet still feminine. She had turned out very well. He laid her head over the side of the tub and began the task of drying her hair. He took the brush from the counter and began working out the knots. Galen enjoyed the sensation of the clean, moist hair being drawn over his fingers and through the brush. The natural wave in her hair began to return as it dried. Galen rose to his feet, lifted her from the tub and carried her to his bed. He laid her gently on one side then walked around to the other. He drew back the covers and reached across to roll her to this side.

Galen carefully positioned Brenda in the bed and pulled the covers over her body. He adjusted the pillow slightly as if to make her more comfortable. Galen sat by her side for a while watching her breathe. The simple rise and fall of her breathing was only made more intriguing by the sheet covering her. He placed his hand between her breasts to feel her heartbeat. The rhythm was slow and easy.

Her hands twitched after nearly half an hour. Her eyes began to move under the lids. Her breathing began to get deeper. Slowly, her eyes opened. Her gaze met by Galen's.

"What happened?" Brenda asked softly.

"I will attempt to explain in a few moments. How do you feel?" Galen leaned over her from the side of the bed. He looked very concerned.

"Were we in an accident?" Brenda's voice grew stronger as her eyes continued to focus on Galen.

"Not exactly, but there have been a few changes. We need to have a long talk."

Chapter Eighteen

The first thing Brenda noticed were her breasts. They remained about the same size they used to be, but they were young. Gravity no longer had any hold over them. They were compact and held their shape as she moved. She looked under the sheet at them in amazement. They sat there firm in their resolution to be noticed. She moved her hand across them, checking if they were real. The sensation told her that they were definitely real and hers. Galen said that he had something to check on and he would be right back. Brenda's curiosity overcame modesty and she pulled the sheet back to expose her naked form. She began rubbing her hands up and down her legs. They felt smooth, even with the fine layer of transparent hair that covered them. Brenda remembered shaving them a few days ago, but the hair had always been coarser than it was now.

She slowly got out of bed. As her feet touched the floor, the sensation shocked her. She could feel the texture of the carpet, not just the softness like before, but she could feel the actual fibers. Carefully, she stood up, a little unsteady at first. She put her hands out to check her balance, and then she took a step. The same thrilling sensation rushed up from her feet with each step. She looked up in the mirror at her reflection. She looked incredible.

Her arms possessed defined muscles as did her legs. She had always had a good body, but nothing like this. She turned to see herself from behind. Even her back had definition, and her behind was as impressive as her breasts. Brenda didn't understand, but for right now, she really didn't care.

Brenda suddenly heard footsteps outside the door. They continued to grow louder. The door should be opening by now. A quick glance in the mirror almost frightened her. She had begun to crouch cat-like. Her new muscle tone becoming even more pronounced. The steps finally stopped. She could hear the sound of the knob being carefully turned. Every nerve on her body stretched to the breaking point.

"Brenda."

The voice had a distorted and dreamy sounding quality against the minute sounds that she had been focusing on. After a second, she finally sorted out that it was Galen.

"Brenda, may I come in?" Galen asked from the door knowing better than to simply walk in.

"Um, yes." She answered, forgetting for the moment that she was nude.

Galen stepped slowly into the room. It appeared as if he was trying not to make any sudden moves. He smiled at her as she rose from her crouched position from in front of the mirror. She stood upright and looked directly at him.

"What happened to me?" Brenda asked in amazement.

Galen didn't answer. Instead, he began to walk around her, admiring her form. The body had an overall lean and powerful looking frame. The legs were well formed, and the feet appeared delicate. The rise and fall of her breathing was smooth and even. The breasts stood at attention as if waiting to be caressed, the neck now lean and sinewy. She had definitely fulfilled his expectations. Oddly, she didn't feel self conscious under his examination. She wasn't sure what she felt. She simply waited for him to finish.

"It is not easy to explain what has happened to you. Come over here, please." Galen finally said as he gestured for her to move closer.

As she stepped towards him, he opened the closet door and removed a silk robe from its hanger. Galen held it open for her to put on. Brenda stepped into the robe. The sensation of the silk rubbing across her body suddenly became the most profoundly erotic experience she had ever had. The muscles under her skin shuddered and jumped at the smooth, cool contact of the exquisite material. She breathed in sharply. She could actually feel his presence. Even with her back to him, she could tell exactly where he stood.

"You have been quite ill for the last couple of days." Galen began.

"What do you mean couple of days? Where am I and what happened to me?" Brenda turned to look him in the eye.

"Do you remember our date?" He asked as he began leading her over to the bed.

"I don't remember very much. It is all still kinda fuzzy." She rubbed a hand across her eyes as she followed him.

Galen had a seat on the end of the bed and guided her down next to him. He turned slightly so that he could face her. "Go ahead and try. Just tell me what you remember."

She nodded her head and looked him directly in the eyes. "Ok, I'll try. I remember the dress. It was very pretty. It was very sweet of you to send it and the limousine. The limousine was good. It was very good. I remember getting out at some building and the moon. The moon was full. It was really too much."

"Go on." Galen prompted.

"I remember you had this room all done up with curtains and candles and wait a minute! There was a fire!" She looked up and down at her body. "I didn't see any burns in the mirror."

"No, you were not burned. While we were, ah, becoming intimate, we apparently had an accident of some type. Candles were knocked over and a small fire was started. I got us out safely. After the fire was out, I saw that you had fallen ill. You had developed a fever. The symptoms were just like a rare virus that I had seen in Europe. I brought you to my home and I have cared for you ever since." Galen almost sounded motherly.

"If I was sick, why didn't you take me to a hospital?"

"A friend of mine is a doctor. I called his office as soon as we arrived. We both agreed on what needed to be done." Galen looked Brenda straight in the eye. He looked very serious. "This is a disease that requires very careful treatment. By the time we convinced one of these American hospitals of what to do, you might have perished and that I would not allow."

Brenda could feel herself falling madly in love with him. How many men would save you from a burning building and nurse you back to health? "But what happened to me?" she asked again looking down at her body.

"The fever causes extreme fluid loss and severe cramping of the muscles. It usually lasts a couple of days. I am told that it is so painful that when you recover you often experience heightened sensitivity. How do you feel?" His dark brown eyes looked apologetic for telling her she might have been in pain.

"I feel fine, I guess." Brenda said thinking about the how the carpet felt when she got out of bed and then the silk robe.

"Good. There is just one other effect the fever leaves you with. Please be careful of your teeth. Because of the severe cramping, you have been gritting your teeth for the last couple of days. Your teeth may be a little worn. I mean that they may be jagged or sharp in a few places. Let me show you. This may look a bit funny, but it could save you from a nasty bite on the tongue." Galen reached into his pocket.

She ran her tongue across the back of her teeth. Now that he had said something about it, they did feel different. As she watched, he pulled two hard rubber dog chew bones from his pocket. These were the type that even the aggressive breeds had to work on for a while before they tore them up. He handed her one as he raised the other to his lips. With almost no effort, he bit the end completely off.

David finally woke up. He experienced a little disorientation so he sat up and looked around for a couple of minutes. He was in a bed, in a house, and wearing new clothes. So, it wasn't some kind of cruel dream. Some rich weirdo wanted to hear about what it was like to be homeless. David figured he had about two months worth of stories to tell. After that, he would just have to make up a few.

He saw the fruit bowl. That hadn't been there when he crawled into bed. At least, he was pretty sure that it hadn't been there. David smiled broadly to himself as he walked over and selected a plum. Room service and everything, this was going to be a sweet gig.

David dropped the slept in clothes in the empty hamper. He didn't even wonder what happened to the old clothes. The whirlpool bath had his undivided attention for now. After the tub filled, he hit the switch that activated the water jets, and lowered himself into the tub. He took his time, enjoying himself immensely. This was the second bath he had taken this year. It felt even better than the first one did yesterday. Today, the water could actually reach him without having to fight its way through the build up of street life.

David spent little time staring into the closet this time. Everything inside looked great. He grabbed a new pair of underwear, gray slacks, and a light blue button-down. He sat down on the end of the bed to tie the laces on the pair of topsiders he had found. He checked himself in the mirror and then walked to the door. With the way things were going right now, he couldn't wait for dinner.

Chapter Nineteen

He knew that David was bathing. He left Brenda to dress for dinner knowing that she would take her time, he also knew that David would not. This posed no problem. Galen knew exactly what he wanted to serve tonight. He had pulled three Cornish hens from the freezer. He had already prepared them to go directly into the oven. Before he had put them in the freezer, he had rubbed them down in butter and French tarragon. Now, all he had to do was unwrap them, put them in the roaster, and set the oven. He placed the makings of a broccoli and rice casserole on the stove and in the steamer.

By the time he could hear David closing his door, the vegetable and cheese tray was on the table with the rest of dinner not far behind.

"How did you sleep?"

The question caught David slightly by surprise. He had just reached the kitchen doorway and hadn't seen or heard anyone yet.

"I feel like I slept for a week. Man, it smells good in here." David answered as he looked greedily into the kitchen.

"Thank you. I don't cook for guests often, so I am showing off a little." Galen said as he continued working at the stove.

"What did you do, spend all day in here or what?" David asked curiously.

"No, I actually pre-pack meals for the freezer. I travel quite a bit, so I rarely have the luxury of taking my time in the kitchen." Galen glanced over his shoulder at David as he answered.

"I never got inta cookin like this. Matter of fact, I hadn't eaten like this in a while." David was obviously interested in everything in the kitchen.

"Well, I am gratified that you are enjoying your stay. My friend will be here this evening to talk with you. Her name is Brenda and she will be joining us for dinner. Would you mind opening the wine?" Galen nodded his head at the bottle and corkscrew on the counter.

"I don't mind at all." David said. He picked up the long, unusually shaped bottle. He looked at the label with its art deco designs. He read the part of the label about the essence of chocolate it was supposed to contain.

"This is a lot better than sleeping in the park." David mused to himself as he worked on getting the cork out of the bottle in one piece. David's mind filled with possibilities. "So, tonight I get to meet this Brenda friend of yours."

As David busied himself with the bottle, Galen studied him closely out of the corner of his eye. The coordination was good, but not great. His scent had cleaned up tremendously. If he didn't know where David had been found, it would have been difficult to tell now. The eyes were no longer bloodshot and the bags underneath them had nearly disappeared. A couple of more days of this type of care and he would probably turn out to be a good-looking man.

Brenda didn't feel like accessorizing as she looked at herself in the mirror again. She twirled to the other side of the mirror, causing the wrap around skirt to swell out slightly with the movement. She debated whether or not to tuck in the pull over sweater or leave it out. Leave it out won the final decision. Galen must keep a lot of extra clothing around the place. Brenda had found the proper size undergarments in the oak dresser by the wall. The skirt and sweater could fit many different sizes because of how they were made. She smiled as she thought of the razzing she was going to give Galen about keeping woman's clothing in the house. She stepped into a pair of black slippers and walked to the door. Brenda just could not get over how good everything felt now. She took a deep breath next to the door as the aroma of poultry and spices reached her. With sudden purpose, she opened the door and walked down the hall towards dinner.

About half way down the hall she stopped. She could hear something strange. Galen was not alone. There was another man in the room with him. She shook her head. How did she know that? She listened again and was slightly startled when she quite distinctly heard the sound of a cork being removed from a bottle of wine.

She continued walking towards the kitchen. The smell of cooking food was absolutely tantalizing. She had always enjoyed the smells of a kitchen, but she had never smelled anything so vibrantly. She could actually taste the air.

As she rounded the corner, Galen began the introductions. "David Langston, I would like you to meet Brenda. Brenda, this is David Langston. He is going to tell us how to survive out on the street. David is homeless."

Other than each other's names, neither of them heard another word Galen had said. David slid beyond the ability to really think clearly. It had been a long time since he had been clean and this close to a woman. When Galen had said something about being studied, he had expected an older more professor type, not this. She looked incredible.

The man's scent commingled with the food. There was something actually palatable about him. Galen was much better looking, but he didn't feel the same as this new man.

"I'm pleased to meet you, David." Brenda said as she stepped forward extending her hand.

David reached out slowly. As their hands touched, they both visibly reacted. It was as if a pleasant electric shock had leapt between them.

She looked directly into his eyes. She could feel herself blush. Brenda found herself nearly overcome by the urge to be very close to this man. She took a deep breath and her manners over came the urges, but she still felt very strangely.

Every little sound seemed magnified. Brenda could hear everything from the faint movements of Galen in the kitchen to the pop of grease from the oven. She thought that she could taste the flavor of the food through the steam in the air. She could almost taste the man in front of her. A faint pounding sounded in her ears. It sounded like a heart beat - David's heart beat.

"Uh, you okay?"

"What? I'm sorry, it's been a strange day." David's question had boomed in her ears, breaking the strange trance that she had been in. This all had caught her quite by surprise.

"Why don't the two of you have a seat at the table, and dinner will be ready in just a moment." Galen said while waving them towards the other room.

David turned in the doorway and led the way to the table. Brenda followed him. She caught herself leering at his backside as he walked. Brenda began to wonder what had come over her. She had been sick for three days and now all she could think about was men.

David was beginning to feel uncomfortable under her gaze. This lady had done nothing but stare. He had begun to feel a little like a goldfish in a bowl.

"Wine?" David offered.

"Yes, thank you."

As David poured the wine into Brenda's glass, he could feel her staring at him again. "Um, Galen says you want to hear about what it's like on the street. You know, as a homeless person." David ventured tentatively.

Brenda really didn't care what they talked about as long as he talked. She was really enjoying listening to his voice. There was something new about how the sound felt in her ears.

"If you would like to talk about it?" She prompted.

"I don't mind." David took a sip of wine then took a deep breath as he looked up and met her eyes. He must be the first homeless person she had ever seen. She was looking straight at him again. David was beginning to fidget under her stare. "I'm not sure where to begin."

"How did you become homeless?" Galen asked from the kitchen.

"I dunno. It just sort of happened. Things just started going bad. Then, one day, I woke up in the park and I've been there ever since. It's not like I planned it or anything." David shrugged his shoulders and took another sip of wine before continuing. "I just barely got the grades to get out of high school. As soon as I got out, me and a few buddies all went to work. We got apartments." David smirked and shook his head. "We got thrown out of apartments, too much partying. We wouldn't show up for work on time or just skip a day here and there. We would get fired and go find new jobs. It was no big deal"

While David talked of jobs, parties, and all the other happenings in his life, Brenda found herself listening to the pattern of the words rather than the content. How he talked had a very set rhythm. The beats in the words told her everything about him. She could tell what he was feeling, not by the look on his face, but by the tones that he used. The longer he talked, the more intently she listened to his body. She could plainly make out the beat of his heart and the rise and fall of his breathing. His clothes made slight rustles as he moved his arms and hands in illustration to his story.

"I hope that everyone is ready to eat." Galen said as he entered the room.

Brenda sat straight back in her chair like a child that had been doing something that she wasn't supposed to do. Galen's voice had broken the trance of David's speaking. Brenda almost looked crossly at Galen for interrupting, but the aroma of the food caught her again. Suddenly, she felt ravenously hungry.

"Man, this looks good. Thanks." David offered as he was handed his plate. He picked up a fork and began without waiting for anyone else.

"Thank you, Galen." Brenda barely said before she followed David's example.

"The bread, I'll be right back." Galen snapped his fingers in remembrance. He smiled broadly to himself as he walked into the kitchen. Everything was going perfectly. David had warmed up nicely.

His story of the streets was actually becoming very interesting. Brenda seemed enthralled. She also looked like she was enjoying her new "side effects". This should prove to be a very interesting evening for everyone.

Galen watched and listened to everything from the kitchen. They both acted just as he had planned. He wasn't sure what exactly would happen next, but he had put all the ingredients together and set them to simmering nicely. He gathered his rolls into a wicker bread server. He carefully folded the cloth over the top and turned to the doorway. He could see that they both subconsciously leaned towards each other. David still talked animatedly between bites. Brenda appeared to be hanging on every word. As Galen entered the room, he flipped back the cloth with the flourish of a waiter in a very expensive restaurant. He extended the basket between the two diners.

"David?" Galen asked as he moved the basket to his side of the table.

"Yeah, thanks. You know, this is really good." David said as he took two rolls from the basket.

"Brenda?" Galen asked as he moved the basket to her side.

"Yes. Thank you." Brenda said as she tore her eyes from David to look at Galen. She blindly took one roll while shifting her intense gaze back to David.

Galen walked to the end of the table and had a seat. He began his own meal as he watched his guests with keen interest. They now lived in their own world, even if they hadn't realized it yet.

Brenda felt like she was approaching sensory overload. Every sound, every scent, and every taste brought her new sensations. She had the feeling of what it would be like for the blind to be seeing perfectly for the first time. She couldn't get over this fascination with David. Every movement he made held her attention. Every sound he made infatuated her. Then the food had arrived and every spice practically sang out to her. The texture of the flesh between her teeth delivered an exquisite sensation. The sound of her teeth scraping lightly on a bone sent shivers down her spine. She even kicked off her shoes so that she could rub her feet across the carpet.

David finished the last morsel on the plate, took a sip of wine, and then he continued, "You know, I guess that is kinda funny. The one job where I don't do nothing wrong. I mean that I had learned my lesson. I didn't go in late. I didn't get in any fights. I didn't even party that much any more. I just go in one morning and there was this bunch of guys running around telling everybody to go home. The company was downsizing and we've been laid off. Laid off, it's a nice way of saying thanks for getting it right and you're fired. I don't know what happened then. A bunch of us went out and got real drunk that afternoon. I don't know what really happened after that. I remember we were gonna drive out to the company office and tell 'em off. I don't remember if we did or didn't." His shoulders slumped as if in defeat. "But I do remember thinking that I couldn't win. Nuthin I ever did turned out right. I think I just gave up."

"My God, that is so sad. It must have been terrible for you." Brenda reached across the table and softly covered David's hand with her own. The touch was so electrifying that they both locked gazes.

Galen had been watching quietly at his end of the table. He smiled to himself knowingly. As their hands touched, he rose, walked up next to David, and picked up the plate and silverware. David barely glanced his direction. Galen continued around the table to Brenda. She glanced up and her lips moved to the word "thanks", but there was no sound. Her attention returned immediately to David. Galen retreated silently to the kitchen. Gently, he placed the dishes in the sink. Forgotten by the two at the table, he walked lightly down the hall to his room. The slight smile that had caressed his lips all evening bloomed into a full grin as he closed his door.

CHAPTER TWENTY

It seemed like they had been talking for hours. David had been telling her about his life on the street. The more he talked, the tighter she held his hand. The part about sleeping alone under a culvert in a park had actually gotten her to begin rubbing his leg with her feet. David just hoped he could keep talking. Tonight was turning out very differently than he had anticipated.

Brenda simply couldn't help herself. Everything this evening was so intense. Walking across carpet barefoot came close to being a sexual experience. Now, the feel of his skin obsessed her. As he told his story, she concentrated on the texture of his palm. There were so many things about a man's hand that she had just never noticed before. She could feel his pulse in his thumb. The center of the palm held tension while the edges were soft. The small hairs on the back of the hand all lay in the same direction.

As Brenda lightly rubbed the skin, she could feel the texture change. The area of skin under her fingertips would warm to the contact. The surface would begin to soften as the capillaries under the skin filled with blood. It utterly amazed her how his skin responded to this light massage. Still holding his hand, she stood up, walked around the table, and took a seat next to him.

David was telling her how they begged for handouts when she got up and moved around next to him. David thought, "Well, it looks like we are gunna talk about this for a while."

He began to tell her how to size up a crowd. David described the way to pick who to approach and how to approach them. He told her what conventions were more generous than others and which ones to avoid all together.

David continued talking while she unbuttoned his sleeve. Gently, she rubbed the exposed skin, enjoying the results. Gradually, she turned the palm up so that she could see the under side of the wrist. She could feel all the muscles and tendons. The veins attracted her attention. They were blue ribbons just under his skin. If she pressed down on one very gently she could feel the warm fluid flowing quickly back to his heart. Brenda could feel the pulse in the arteries buried deeper in his flesh. His pulse grew stronger and quicker. She rubbed further up the forearm. As she did this, she could feel his pulse quicken more. She could see the blood swelling the veins.

David began to sweat. He looked around for Galen. He expected him to reappear at any moment. Things like this just didn't happen.

David continued to tell Brenda about a convention that had been very generous to the panhandlers, but he was having trouble concentrating. He looked around again and realized that they were truly alone. Brenda was utterly captivated by his arm and actually had not been listening to a word he said for some time. David let the story die off as he began to really enjoy Brenda's exploration of his arm.

She slowly lowered her head for a closer look. Brenda didn't notice that David had stopped talking and was just enjoying her attentions. At an impulse, she touched the end of her tongue to the skin of his wrist. David moaned and shivered at the touch. He placed his other hand on her shoulder. The taste exploded all along her tongue. She could taste far more than she ever dreamed. Brenda could actually taste how he felt. His skin was slightly salty and moist. She could taste the heat rising in his body. David simply couldn't believe what was happening, but he wasn't about to stop it. He hadn't been on the streets that long.

"Brenda, let's go back to my room, okay?" He whispered hopefully.

Brenda answered by gracefully rising to her feet and allowing him to escort her down the hall. David opened the door and guided her into the room. Still holding hands, David was forced to turn to let her pass. This made the whole maneuver look and feel like a dance step. He closed the door then she pulled him over to the bed. He followed her unable to do anything else.

When they reached the side of the bed, she turned his back to the bed and pushed him down.

David was in too much shock to realize that she had actually lifted him from the floor. His mind was having enough trouble dealing with the last two days to notice small details like that. He moved up in the bed to make room for her.

Brenda pounced onto the edge and pursued her quarry to the head of the bed. She pulled his hands away from the buttons on his shirt. She was in control and she was determined to keep it that way. She very slowly, teasingly, unbuttoned the shirt and slid it off his shoulders. He leaned forward to help. When the shirt reached his wrists, Brenda shoved him back, trapping his hands in the sleeves of the shirt. He didn't seem to be protesting his confinement, so she continued.

Tentatively, she kissed his shoulder. She could taste everything. The salt, his lust, and even his disbelief, all had different flavors. She began to run her tongue over every square inch of skin. David moaned and threw his head back.

"Oh my, God. I don't believe this." He gasped.

Brenda paid no attention to him. This was for her not him. She worked her way to his nipples. She had become completely engrossed in how they reacted to her. She suddenly leaned back and pulled her sweater off over her head. The sweater was thrown off the bed followed by the bra.

Brenda began to rub David's chest with one hand and her own with the other. With each hand, she circled a nipple. As the sensation traveled across her, she could see the same happening to David. She traded to the other side of each of them. As she caressed, the nipples became hard and erect. Satisfied that they were both having the same feelings, she returned her full attention to David. She massaged his chest with both hands. She carefully guided her tongue across his collarbone and up to the soft flesh above. David tilted his head back to allow her full access. Brenda could feel his pulse just under his skin. The sensation fascinated her. She covered his throat with her mouth. She could taste his very life like this.

Almost reluctantly, Brenda began to move back down to his chest and gradually to his abdomen. As she bent to her work, David's gaze became fixed on the wonderful breasts standing majestically out from her body. She pulled her hands powerfully across his ribs in time to his breathing. His breath moved like a bellows, deep and rhythmic.

Brenda rose up and turned around to face his feet. While she settled down, straddling him, he freed his hands from the shirt restraint. Brenda undid the leather laces of the topsiders. She had begun to pull them off when she arched back as if stung. David had reached forward and begun to rub her back. The motion of his fingers against her muscles caused her to have a small wave of sensations sweep across her. Warmth flooded between her thighs as her back danced with pleasure. She remembered to inhale after the waves of pleasure had begun to pass. She allowed him to continue stroking her back while she got herself back under as much control as she could. She gripped David's feet and applied pressure until she heard him moan loudly.

"Damn that feels good."

To her surprise, the toes and feet responded just like the hands. As she caressed them, she could feel the texture change. Brenda had never realized how similar the hands and feet actually were. She was becoming impatient to discover more, but everything seemed to demand her attention.

David began to rub strongly on the small of her back and across the firm buttocks facing him. The first time he reached her thigh, more waves of pleasure washed across her. As the last wave passed, Brenda stood up next to the bed. She gave David a long look as his eyes bounced back and forth between her eyes and her breasts.

"Well, go for it." David finally said as the suspense became too much for him.

She reached over to undo the buckles and zipper that kept him confined. David watched the action not sure what he was supposed to do now. Nothing had gone the way he had expected for the last two days. He didn't think that it was going to start now.

He rose up to allow her to pull the clothing down his legs. As she lifted his underwear away from the skin, he moaned at the feeling of being free. The clothing had become very restrictive. Brenda threw them to the floor and gave David another good long look.

"Well, come on." David prompted.

A moment later, she had left her clothing on the floor. Brenda climbed back into the bed and shoved David back down onto his back. She started massaging his legs. This had become more than David could bear. His system was beginning to overload. He tried to sit back up and reach for Brenda. She shoved him roughly back down. She could feel the heat and the throbbing. She was not ready to lose him yet.

She grabbed him roughly and pressed firmly with her thumb just below the head. The shock alone was enough for David to lose the immediacy of his need. He just lay there and stared into her eyes. He had finally accepted that she was in total control.

Brenda leaned over and kissed his thigh. The muscle jumped as if burned. She applied more consistent pressure with her mouth. She worked her way up the thigh, slowly. A wildness entered David's eyes as he sat up again. Curiously, anywhere she touched with her tongue felt slightly cool. If he had been paying attention, he would have noticed a slight numbness. She didn't shove him back down this time. He began to caress her back and neck. Brenda could feel a great need building in her. Part of the need was beginning to cry out for release. The rest felt like a great thirst that hadn't been sated.

Brenda's ears were filled with a distant roaring sound and her need had become unbearable. Gently, she kissed her way up his body until she had him straddled. His eyes snapped open and met her gaze. They both repositioned each other slightly before Brenda leaned back slowly. They both gasped as the tip touched the edge of her opening. Both trembling, they supported each other as she began to bear down. She was ready to accept him. The curious coolness allowed David to withstand the warm, rich friction of penetration. They both held their breath as she completed her descent. She rose to take her weight onto her knees. David looked down her body. He looked over the breasts begging for attention as he struggled to a sitting position.

Brenda set the rhythm. David supported her as she swung her legs around him. Fully embraced, the rhythm quickly reached a fevered pitch. The heat and fullness of him inside her had a greater intensity than any other sensation she had ever felt. She could feel his firmness increase. His thigh muscles began to tense. Her own deep pleasure had already begun, slowly at first, growing more intense with each thrust deep inside her. Brenda could hear his pulse quite loudly now. Each thrust was harder and more desperate than the last. She became overcome as she buried her head into the hollow of his neck. Suddenly, the need was all that existed. Her need consumed her utterly. She felt life itself flooding into her. Her mouth was filled with his essence.

Her legs gripped so tightly around David's back that they began to cramp. His firmness exploded in liquid heat. Each thrust was volcanic. A final spasm throughout his body was all she remembered before she passed out.

Chapter Twenty One

The dreams were the dreams of decadent royalty, water and fire, screaming and laughter, images flashed and rolled throughout her sleep. No matter how bizarre or disturbing the scene, she couldn't wake up. She tossed and turned, fighting the sheets. She kept patting around the bed, looking for something. Somewhere in her mind, she remembered that she wasn't supposed to be alone. Brenda eventually captured the spare pillow and hugged it tightly to her. She finally settled down to a deep sleep.

Hours later, Brenda slid out of bed and nearly had to crawl to the bathroom. Her legs felt rubbery. She rubbed and shook her head the whole trip. It felt like it had been stuffed with cotton, stomped down, and packed again. She had never had a hangover like this. When she made it back to bed, she tried to sort out what happened last night. After a couple of minutes of concerted effort, her memory began to work shakily. She looked under the covers. She was naked. Her eyes opened a little wider as she recognized that relaxed feeling between her legs.

"Well, it's pretty obvious that I slept with someone last night," Brenda concluded out loud. The thought that she slept with someone jerked her a little more awake. The name David came to mind, but she remembered something about his being homeless. None of this made sense. Frustrated, she got back up and walked to the bathroom. The sensation of the carpet under her bare feet was still incredible. She stopped in the doorway as her foot touched the cool tile. This being hyper sensitive had something to do with last night, but it wasn't registering yet. She began to feel like she really needed a shower.

She stepped into the misty stream of water. The touch of the water droplets sent shivers throughout her body. Brenda picked up the bar of soap and wet it between her hands. Once the lather gathered, she began down one leg. As her hands rubbed up and down the calf, she looked more closely at the muscle. She flexed her foot downward and an Olympic quality muscle smoothly rippled. This began to feel like déjà vu. She remembered that Galen had said something about her being sick. She couldn't think of any disease that left you looking like this. Galen, the name floated around in her head for a second. Big date, lots of candles, and dinners, but not whom she slept with last night. That thought was not a good one. This was his house, that was his bed, and she had slept with David the homeless person.

Brenda quickly finished the shower and toweled off. She didn't notice how well her body had finished developing. Yesterday, she had been impressed; today she would have been amazed. The musculature had grown more cut and mature. Her mind was elsewhere.

She grabbed a black jumpsuit out of the closet and slipped into it. She forgot to put on any shoes. Her dream was disturbing her now. Something about all of this wasn't right. She felt like her mind refused to tell her something that she needed to know. It was time to find Galen and start asking a few questions.

"How are you doing this evening?"

Brenda was startled as the voice greeted her before she had reached the door. She stepped through the doorway and peered in. Galen sat behind his desk putting away business papers.

"How did you sleep?" Galen asked a second question, still fishing for an answer.

"Um, fine I guess. What time is it?" Brenda asked as she looked around. She didn't remember this room.

"It is about seven in the evening. I was just about to fix dinner." Galen explained as he put both hands on the top of the desk.

"Will David be with us tonight?" She asked already afraid of the answer.

"Oh, I doubt very severely if he will be joining us ever again." Galen looked almost amused as he answered. His eyes danced with secrecy.

The dreams and a feeling of dread overcame her. Galen didn't look upset and that really scared her. All the men she knew wouldn't be this calm if their date had slept with the house guest.

"What, um, happened to David?" Brenda ventured carefully.

"Don't you remember?" Galen paused for a moment then continued, "You killed him last night."

The flat, matter-of-fact way in which he spoke ripped into her soul. Her knees turned to jelly and her head began to swim. She collapsed into the chair on her side of the desk. She couldn't believe what he just said; yet somehow, it sounded true. His words burst the wall that she had put up in her mind. The memories came flooding back. Her tears began to flow. She balled up into the chair in complete disbelief. Galen didn't try to console her. He didn't even look up from his work on the desk. He waited for her to calm down. He knew better than to interfere with her emotions right now.

After he had cleared most of the paperwork from the top of the desk, he looked up at Brenda. She had finally begun to unball herself.

"What have you done to me?" She asked quietly while looking at her hands. No answer, he just sat there and looked at her.

"What have I done?" She pleaded, looking him in the eyes.

"You have done what you must do to survive. Nothing more, nothing less." He waited for the next question.

"What do you mean survive?" Brenda asked truly confused.

"How old do you think I am?" Galen answered her question with a question.

"I don't give a damn how old you are. I want to know...."

Loudly, Galen cut her off, "I am," then softly, "far older than your grandparents. Now, ask me how."

"Ok, how?" she quipped shortly. She turned in the chair to face him.

"By surviving on the lives of others." Galen's expression changed from deadpan to that of an instructor. He continued, "at least once a month, we must augment our diet with the living or we will cease to exist."

"What the hell are you talking about?" The edge of panic crept into her voice.

Galen stood up and walked around the desk to the front. He sat on the edge of the desk like a schoolteacher getting comfortable for a lecture. "I was born human just like you. I was a child, and I grew up to become a young man in my village. While hunting one day, it became late and as the sunset faded, I became the hunted. An *upir* tried to claim me as her trophy. I survived or so I thought. Wounded and exhausted, I managed to make it back home before I fell ill with the same fever that you contracted from me. I went through the same process that you have just gone through. It is called rebirth because you are reborn as an *upir*. You have become more than human." Galen stood up and began to pace as he continued, "Look at yourself. Don't you feel the very air around you? Can't you hear the faintest sound? Look at the new musculature that you possess. Age has faded from your body. You feel strong." Galen stared at his own hands as they curled into fists and the forearms flexed. "You have been given the ability to defeat age for a while. You do not have to worry about running out of time."

Brenda's eyes met his as she tried desperately to understand. "What are you talking about? What did you mean I killed somebody last night."

"I will make it simpler for you. You have inherited from me several very unique abilities. I have given you a new type of life, the life of the *upir*. We are stronger and faster than we were as simple humans. We also live much longer than humans. As a matter of fact, we provide a service for the humans. We are their predators." Galen's eyes were wide with fascination as his hands moved with every point he made.

"What am I? Some kind of vampire, or something undead, or some bullshit like that?" Brenda could feel anger rising up inside her.

"If you are asking me if you fed on the man from last night. The answer is yes. As you gave him something he wanted, you took what you needed to survive, his life." Galen calmly explained.

The answer hit her like a blow. That night with Galen had been no date. He was not being romantic. Her sexual favors had not been the dessert. She had been the main course. He had

169

given her nothing, but lies. That same feeling that had overcome her last night, screamed in rage in her mind. An immense beast rushed her and took her body from her control. She had never felt this furious before. The part of her mind that was Brenda simply sat down out of the way of this new part of her.

Galen knew she would respond sooner or later. Most females liked to throw things and scream. He assumed the Brenda would be that type. She caught him off guard.

He was standing there. His lips were moving, but she had ceased to hear anything, but the beast in her soul scream. Brenda lunged from the chair straight into his chest. The impact lifted him from the ground. They hurtled backwards into the wall. There was a burst of white dust and a loud cracking sound as they exploded through the wall into the hallway. Galen landed hard and flat. A ripping sensation across the small of his back told him that he was in real trouble.

Galen tried to breathe but he couldn't. Brenda crouched in the center of his chest where she landed, her hands frozen around his neck. The opening of his eyes enraged her further. Keeping her grip on his neck, Brenda planted her feet on the floor. She stood up hauling Galen from the ground like so much dead weight. He grabbed her arms to pull them from his neck. She slammed his head back into the wall behind him. More white dust flew up into the air as his head shattered the drywall. His arms gripped her again. His eyes met hers. He could see that she had given completely over to the fury. She screamed in primal rage as she spun out into the hallway. Halfway through the spin, she lowered her hips and whipped her arms over her head to the front. Galen was wrenched from the wall and flung over Brenda's head. He crashed to the floor over ten feet away. He looked like twisted wreckage against the wall.

Through the red curtain of rage, Brenda could see his twisted body crumpled at the end of the hallway. The runner rug had pulled up from the carpet. Chunks of drywall fell everywhere. The dust was nearly blinding. There were blood spatters along Galen's flight path.

Curiously, even though he hadn't moved, the fact that he still breathed kept her enraged. She stormed towards him to end this. If she needed to feed, he might make a good place to start. The deceitful bastard did this to her and now he was going to pay for it.

Brenda never saw the movement of Galen's leg as it lashed out. He kicked her viciously in the ankles as she stepped into range. Her legs slapped together, and she dropped like a stone, face first to the floor. At the last possible moment, she caught her weight on her hands. His other foot landed on the back of her head just as she caught herself. The impact drove her forehead into the floor like a spike. Pain exploded behind her eyes.

It had been a very long time since anything, or anyone had challenged him physically. Trevor had been a hungry fool looking for any opportunity.

He had been easy to dispose of. Galen had been over confident with Brenda. She was already much stronger than he had anticipated. She had inflicted a great deal of damage very quickly. Her instincts were perfect for her new life. He wasn't going to give her the moment to recover that she had mistakenly given him. Galen hammered his fingers into the wall and pulled himself to his feet. His back screamed in agony at every movement.

He reached down, grabbed her by her hair, and hauled her up. His pain showed plainly on his face.

"Nice start." He growled. He struck her in the ribs so hard that she collapsed back to the floor.

Galen lifted her from the ground by her hair again and hurled her down the hall. She hit hard, but spun around to her feet. Crouched like a lioness about to charge, Brenda glared at Galen.

He couldn't make it to her in time to stop her so he would have to make her come to him. His voice rose commanding, "You are too young to defeat me. On your knees and beg my forgiveness and I..."

Brenda rushed him. He tried to drive her down to the floor, but his back didn't have the strength. She slammed into his mid-section forcing him back into the wall. Galen snarled as he hit on his back again. He shot an elbow into her back. Her knees buckled under the impact, for a moment. She shoved her way back up to a standing position. Galen ducked as she slashed at his eyes. Wall paper shredded under her nails as they passed. Galen punched at her head with all his might. Brenda had to step back to avoid the blow.

They glared at each other. Galen, grateful for the few seconds of reprieve from the combat, breathed deeply. This had to end soon. Brenda stepped forward. Galen lashed out at the movement. She leaned back out of the blow's way. Galen lunged forward at her. She caught his hands and retreated back a few steps. Galen shoved her back as hard as he could. He now had enough room to work with.

"You will have to do better than that to kill me, child." Galen said coldly, heavily accenting the word child. He laughed a cold hollow laugh.

His laughter was more than she could bear. Brenda leapt at him. She was going to enjoy ripping him to pieces. He waited to move until she was just about to make contact. His right arm swatted her outstretched hands upwards as he twisted his body savagely to the right. His back protested, but held. The left arm held rigid like a steel pipe smashed into her sternum. The impact and her momentum flung her into the air like a marionette ripped from its strings. She landed hard. Brenda lay dazed by the dual impacts. Her head swam. She couldn't focus on her target for just a moment.

No sooner had she hit the floor than Galen had jerked her up by the hair.

"You WILL learn your place." His voice was more a growl than words. He slapped Brenda so hard her legs gave out. He hauled her up again.

"You will not challenge me again." He slapped her again. Again, she collapsed only to be hauled up once more. He could see that most of the fight was knocked out of her. Most was not enough.

"Have you learned?" He asked in a conversational tone. Just as her eyes focused, he struck her in the ribs just under the breast. She dropped to her knees. He pulled her up again. He looked into her eyes again.

"Have you learned?" He asked again calmly. She couldn't breathe. Her eyes rolled wildly. He slapped her again. She bounced off the door facing and fell toward Galen. He caught her hair and kept her upright. Her arms and legs hung limply.

"Have you learned?" He asked slowly this time. He already knew the answer. He wasn't really disturbed that it took this kind of treatment, but he knew if he didn't win now she would kill him, soon. Her throat was exposed as she hung there. Galen knew that he should take her now, but for some reason he didn't feel like it. Besides, she showed such great potential.

Utterly defeated, the beast meekly said, "Yes."

Both Brenda and the beast in her mind blissfully passed out.

Chapter Twenty Two

"Day four. Four days. Haven't they heard of overnight delivery in London?" Maggie sourly thought out loud as she looked at her desk pad calendar. She hadn't been very patient this week. Friday had now arrived and she had only grown more and more restless as the week progressed. She had to know if her suspicions were right. The daily couriers to the office had begun to look at her like she was crazy. Every time something came in, she literally ran over to see what it was.

Maggie, Tina, and Morley had gone through all of the Mircalla files with a fine tooth comb. Mr. Mircalla had a lot of transactions, in fact, far too many transactions for his type of business. He moved a lot of money around and not all of it made sense, but they couldn't find anything illegal. Morley thought Mr. Mircalla was just trying to hide stuff from ex-wives or something like that. Tina just thought that all this intrigue was exciting. Rob thought she was obsessing a little bit over that ring.

The courier came through the door with two white boxes marked with overseas stickers. Maggie barely resisted the urge to tackle the man. Calmly, she stood up and walked over.

"I think I have those boxes you've been looking for." He said with a smile. "Sign on 18 and 19, please."

She took the clipboard and signed it quickly. She smiled broadly as she returned it. "Thanks. These are the ones."

Maggie picked up both boxes and headed straight for her desk. She set the heavy boxes down and reached for her letter opener to split open the packing tape. She flipped through the top couple of inches of paperwork. This was exactly what she had been looking for. She looked at the monitor and keyboard on the desk. This was going to be a lot of work. Maggie pursed her lips as she changed her mind. They had not been hired to audit his accounts, therefore, no reason to punch all this in. Even if Tina helped, it would take a week. She needed to spread this stuff out and find one month in particular.

She stood up, walked over to the conference room, and looked inside. The room was empty.

"Good." She said to herself as she stepped back out into the hallway. Maggie turned abruptly when she suddenly felt the shock of a squirt of cold water strike her in the middle of the back.

"All right, Rob, you got me. Now, come give me a hand." Maggie surrendered with a purpose. She didn't have time for games right now.

"What? Those boxes finally come in." Rob asked with interest. She ignored him as she walked back over to her desk. He followed her obediently. Rob was curious about what she had waited so impatiently for all week.

"Grab those boxes and take them to the conference room for me." She smiled at him innocently and added, "Please."

"That's right, I'm not too bright, but I carry stuff real good, uh?" He teased.

"Thank you." She said as she picked up her coffee cup and went for a refill. Rob had disappeared before she got to the conference room. She sat down and began to sort out the files. They had already been sorted into manila folders labeled by month and year. It only took her a few minutes to find the proper month.

Maggie removed the rubber band on the folder and spread out the contents. She carefully sorted the sheets of information into related piles. She read over the recap of the month and just like she expected, all of the transactions had been lumped under general accounts. Whoever had processed all this had done a good job; they just didn't have much inclination to research every detail. A pattern leapt up from the page at her. She had seen this exact same transaction pattern earlier when Morley had spread out Mircalla's current accounts.

Maggie stopped sorting and held her breath. The copy she had in her hand was the one piece of information she had been looking for. It was a recap of his travel activities taken from his credit card receipts. Mr. Mircalla had been in town the night Jean and Steve disappeared. She had never met Jean's date for that night, but Jean had talked about him a lot the week before she disappeared. Jean had called him Galen. Maybe that "G" in his name stood for Galen. According to Jean, her date traveled a lot, seemed very cultured, spoke with a pronounced accent, and he had this incredible ring that he wore. Mr. Mircalla even fit the physical description down to the brown eyes. Tears began to well up in the corners of Maggie's eyes. She set that piece down by itself. With hands nearly shaking, she continued sorting the rest of the month. A couple of reports later, she found a copy of a credit card statement showing a couple of large cash withdrawals on the day her friends had disappeared.

Maggie understood that all of this was nothing more than circumstantial evidence. If Morley had been right about all of this activity being done to hide something, then she was afraid that Mr. Mircalla might have had something to do with what happened to Jean. She remembered the pattern that they had discovered in his travel plans. She slid everything that had to do with invoicing to the side. She was after his personal travel.

There were two business trips to the same place in California that month. She tossed those in the pile on the table. She finally found the other two trips. Just like she thought, they went to different cities. She walked quickly to the copier. Halfway there, she saw Tina walking straight up to her.

"Rob said the boxes were here." Tina's eyes were open wide with curiosity.

"I already have them in the conference room. Would you shoot me a copy of these and bring them to me?" Maggie asked with more composure than she felt.

"You bet." Tina answered as she grabbed the papers from Maggie's hand. Maggie turned and walked straight back to the conference room. Tina hurried to the copier. She tried to read the pages as she walked.

Maggie sipped her coffee while she rebundled the papers on the table back into the manila folder. She set the stack in the chair next to her and picked up the previous month. She closed her eyes and took a deep breath. She exhaled slowly and opened her eyes as she opened the folder. Within two pages, the pattern had already become apparent.

"Here you go." Tina announced as she entered the room.

"Great. Hand me the copies and put the originals back in the file." Maggie pointed to the chair then continued, "Sort that one back into order for me, thanks."

Tina picked up the file from the chair and took it to the end of the oblong table. Maggie was taking apart the next file. She knew exactly what she was looking for. She perused the recaps to confirm that the pattern was still there. It was. There was the travel recap and just like she thought, two of the trips were business, two were personal. She set the business receipts down and read the remaining. One trip here and one trip to Jackson confirmed her suspicions. Maggie could see Tina closing the first manila folder.

"Okay, we need a copy of this." Maggie said as she held out the papers in her hands.

"All right, be right back." Tina took the papers and walked out the door.

Maggie picked out the month after Jean's disappearance. She already knew what she would find, but she had to confirm it. She skipped the recaps and dug for the travel receipts. She leaned back heavily in her chair as she read. There were four trips, just like always. Two of them were business, and two of them were not. None of them were here. One business trip went to California, the other, to Las Vegas. The first personal trip returned to Jackson and it featured the expected large cash withdrawal. The other trip went to Canton, a new city in the rotation.

Tina walked in with the copies and stopped when she saw the look on Maggie's face. "Are you okay?"

"Yeah, I'm fine. Here are the last ones we need a copy of." She handed the papers to Tina and accepted the papers that she held. While Tina made another trip to the copier, Maggie began closing up the files. She was thinking furiously. She had established that he had been in town at the time of Jean's disappearance, but what did that prove? There were a lot of people in town that week. She shook her head. Maybe Rob was right. Perhaps, she was just obsessing over Jean's death because she didn't want to believe another friend had killed her dearest friend.

"Here you go. Now what?" Tina asked excitedly as she reappeared at the door.

Maggie looked at her watch, then at Tina. "We straighten this stuff up. Then we go grab Rob and make him take us to an early lunch."

They picked up a couple of other early lunch goers and went across the street for barbecue. Everyone did the best they could not to wear too much of lunch back with them. The conversation stayed light, leaving Maggie grateful for the distraction from her own dark thoughts.

When they returned to the office, the interns had delivered the mail and picked up the completed files. Maggie sorted through her allocation the day's mail. Unexpectedly, she had received a business tax bill for Mircalla Enterprises. Maggie had always heard that timing was every thing, now she had absolute proof it happened. The postal service and fate had just given her a perfect excuse, to do exactly what she wasn't sure, but she wasn't going to waste this golden opportunity.

She rang the intercom to the intern's cubicle. "Michelle, I need a letter of authorization for business taxes for a new client. I have the original form at my desk."

"Yes Ms. DeVane, I'll be right there." The young voice responded.

A few minutes later, a young lady walked by and picked up the folder Maggie had laid in the "out" tray. Maggie looked through the information in the client database on Mr. Mircalla. Maggie was a little surprised to see that he had a local phone number because she remembered that he had flown in for the meeting. This made her more determined than ever. Her eyebrows knitted close together as she pulled up a reverse lookup web site. She clicked through a couple of windows and waited as the computer looked for a match. A few seconds later and she had what she wanted, his address.

Chapter Twenty Three

He thought he heard the phone ring. Slowly, he opened his eyes. The phone rang in the study again. Galen painfully sat up in bed. His back felt like it was on fire. The back of his head pounded in rhythm to his heartbeat. The phone persistently rang again. Tenderly, he rose to his feet, the sheet sliding off his nude body. He interlaced his fingers, stretched his arms over his head, and arched his back. Slowly, he increased the arch to an impossible angle until he heard several loud pops of protest from his spine. He leaned forward to touch his toes. After holding that position for a couple more rings of the phone, he pressed his palms to the floor without bending his knees.

Galen grabbed the backs of his legs, and pressed his chest against his thighs. He stood back up and reached for his robe. The robe covered his magnificently muscular and lean body. It also covered huge purple and blue area across the small of his back.

He turned back to the bed and tenderly pulled the covers over Brenda's shoulder. She would sleep for a while longer. The phone finally stopped ringing. Galen walked out the door and down the hall. As he approached the office, the extent of the damage caused during last night's "exchange" became very apparent. The walls had been gouged in places. In a few other places, no wall remained and the timbers had been shattered. Wood fragments and chunks of drywall had been scattered everywhere. The dust had settled on everything. Galen carefully stepped through the devastation that had once been a hallway and into the study. Except for the dust and the gaping hole in the wall, the room was in relatively good shape.

He opened a drawer in the credenza and pulled out a dusting rag. He sat down after wiping out the chair and began cleaning the desk. Brenda's purse from a few nights ago still sat on the corner. He patted the drywall dust off of it and set it back on the desk. Galen pressed his lips tightly together as he looked around. He really had other things to do today, but house repairs would have to be done first.

The phone rang again. Galen, annoyed at the interruption, answered in a voice that gave no indication of his mood. "Hello, may I help you?"

Maggie nearly lost her nerve. His voice sounded so soft and pleasant with that odd accent. "May I speak to Mr. Mircalla, please?"

"Speaking"

"Mr. Mircalla, this is Margaret DeVane with Lawson Accounting. Um, I would like to talk with you, if you have a moment."

Galen's mind rushed back to the dinner meeting and ran a quick memory check of the attendees. In an instant, he had a visual memory of her. "Ms. DeVane, what can I do for you today?"

Maggie suddenly felt like she was lost in a dark closet. She felt unsure of herself or what to say. "Please call me Maggie. Everyone else does." She said stalling.

"In that case, Maggie. Please call me Galen." He hesitated as he heard something like a gasp from the other end of the phone.

Maggie covered her mouth with her hand. She had been right, the accent, the ring, and now, the name all matched. It was too late for Maggie to back off now. Caught off balance by his name, she completely forgot about the pretense of the business tax form. "Actually sir, um, Galen. I didn't call you about business. It's actually a personal matter."

All of Galen's internal warning signals went off in his head, but instinctively, he knew that he had already blundered, nothing to do now but press on. "Yes. Please continue."

"Do you remember someone by the name of Jean Talbot?"

Galen could hear the tightening of the breath on the other end. It was too late to use a cover story. He had planned on leaving soon. Now, it looked like his departure would be sooner that he had planned. First, he would have to do something about this one. She carried memories that could prove to be very dangerous.

"It would have been about five years ago." She added.

"Here in town?" Galen asked.

The voice sounded hopeful. "Yes."

Galen made up his mind quickly. It was as good a time as any to show Brenda the wonders of the rest of the world. They would leave as soon as he cleaned up a few loose ends. He might as well put this Maggie into the exit strategy.

"Yes, I remember Jean. It was an absolute tragedy what happened." The tone in his voice sounded sad as he went on. "I had only known Jean a short time. I travel quite a bit in my line of work as I am sure that you are aware."

"Yes." She prompted in his pause.

"She was a bright and wonderful woman. As a matter of fact, we were supposed to meet for drinks the night the police say she disappeared. I had a meeting run late that night. I called her, but got no answer. She never showed up at my hotel. It was a few weeks later that I saw in the newspaper that her ex-boyfriend had been found dead and the authorities presumed that he had killed Jean and then himself."

The voice that Maggie listened to over the phone had been falling off into saddened gasps and finally had become overcome with emotion as the words tumbled out.

"I apologize, Maggie, but I have often wondered, if my meeting hadn't run late - would Jean be alive today? It has been a while since I have spoken to anyone about this. It is simply too painful."

"I'm sorry to put you through this, Galen. It's just that when I saw you at dinner last week, you looked exactly like Jean's descriptions. I knew that it had to be you." Maggie felt vindicated in her suspicions, but she wasn't going to let this bastard know it.

She knew too much. Galen knew that he needed to do something about her immediately. The past month had just not been going his way. Galen grimaced as he remembered the van that had been hunting Trevor, the fire, and now, the accounting firm in London had released records to this new firm. A firm that just so happened to employ a woman who, by some dark chance, remembered him from five years ago. Galen shook his head in frustration. He needed to go back to the places in this world where life was simpler, and the people more superstitious. This country was closing in on him from all directions.

"Maggie, this may sound like a strange question, but would you like to have lunch next week. I would rather talk about Jean, well, face to face. I find the telephone to be too impersonal for this kind of conversation. There are so many things I would like to ask you." Galen sounded very sincere.

The sadness and longing behind the words pulled at her heart in spite of her suspicions. "I

187

would love to sit down with you and tell you about Jean. I even have the newspaper clippings about all this," she paused, "if you would like to see them?"

"I would be forever grateful. Are you free for Monday?" Galen sounded almost hopeful.

"Not really for lunch. How about after work?" Maggie asked as she looked over at her desk calendar.

"That would actually be much better for me. Shall I meet you at the office?" Galen sounded relieved.

"That would be fine. I'll see you Monday at five." Maggie agreed.

"I will be there Maggie. Thank you so much for calling and talking with me. I am looking forward to Monday."

"Thank you Galen. I'll see you then. Good bye."

"Good bye, Maggie." He said as he placed the phone on the hook. He opened the top desk drawer and removed a black credit card file. He paged through it rapidly then picked up the phone again. Monday would be fine. That was plenty of time to arrange his travel plans and her disappearance. He never truly settled into one place completely and he had just moved in here a short time ago. He would be ready to leave in just a few short hours.

Maggie leaned forward and tapped the intercom, "Michelle, do you have that authorization ready for me?"

"Yes ma'am.   I'll bring it right over."   She responded cheerily.

Something important felt like it was about to fall in place. Maggie knew that the missing pieces in Jean's disappearance somehow were with Galen. She didn't know how she knew, but she had a gut feeling she couldn't ignore. She stared at the business form like it held a secret. Maggie shook it slightly and laid it on the desk.

"Monday's great, but you're going to see me in about an hour, Mr. Terrance Galen Mircalla, and you're going to tell me why Jean is dead." Maggie said out loud to herself.

CHAPTER TWENTY FOUR

Brenda heard the phone ring and didn't care. She felt him get out of bed. She heard him moan slightly when he stretched. She allowed herself to slip back into the dreams of the decadent. She really didn't want to wake up. This week had simply been too much for anyone to comprehend. Last week, her life had been up and down just like anybody else's. This week, her life had turned its back on reality and now pursued some kind of fever dream.

She heard Galen come back into the room. The closet door opened and she heard the rustle of clothing. Brenda felt his presence as he leaned over her and kissed her lightly on the cheek. He whispered that he had to leave, but he would be back soon. She didn't respond. She didn't even bother to move for a great while, but her mind drifted into activity. She began to recap the last few weeks in her mind.

She had a great date with this incredible guy that hadn't even made a pass at her. She got a new dress, a ride in a limo, and some chocolate covered strawberries. Then, mister wonderful went down on her and tried to kill her. Instead of dying, she contracted vampirism from the guy, and to think, she used to worry about venereal diseases. Next, she spent a few days in a coma becoming an upir or something like that. The first day awake, Galen lied to her about everything. Then, she had dinner with a homeless guy named David. She nearly raped the guy at the dinner table and finally killed him in bed. Admittedly, he should have been smiling but he was still dead. Galen must have hidden the body while she slept. She woke up and Galen told her the truth. She didn't like the truth so she tried to rip his head off, literally. Oh yeah, she now had the body of a twenty-year-old track star.

She rolled over and moaned audibly. She'd had enough of the thoughts running through her head. One other thing, that great new body had a lot of new bruises. Galen didn't like having her try to rip his head off and he let her know this in no uncertain terms. Then, he turned back into the great guy again. He fed her dinner and then explained all about her new life. A couple of facts that stood out was that they were very strong and very hard to kill. They seemed to live for a very long time as long as they fed. They had to have living blood about once a month or so. If they didn't feed on a timely basis they would age quickly and very painfully. Eventually, the lack of feeding would force them to become something he called a revenant. She had been very tired, so they had gone to bed, his bed. He undressed her and put her under the covers. He got undressed and climbed in with her. All either of them did was fall deeply to sleep, side by side.

As Brenda sat up slowly, the sheet slid off. All of this mess floating in her brain had to be some kind of nightmare. She moved. The pain from the bruises tried to tell her that this had been no dream. She walked gingerly over to the mirror. She possessed a real good knot on her forehead at the hairline. The bruises around her ribs glowed in a vibrant blend of blue and purple. She turned and looked down the other side. Without the bruises, she had an incredible body. Even the small lines on her face that had begun to sneak in a few birthdays ago had vanished. She didn't really look younger, just better. Brenda opened the closet and clothes were already hanging there for her. Somehow, she knew that they would be there. A pair of blue jeans and a pull over would do for now. Gradually, she wandered out into the hall. She rounded the corner in the hallway and stopped. She had to admit that the amount of damage she had caused was impressive. The place was destroyed. When she reached the hole in the study wall, she was amused to see that the desk and chair were absurdly clean.

Brenda had been too preoccupied to notice much the last time she had been in the study, but her purse sat on the corner of the desk. She picked it up and opened it. The purse made all the rest of the surroundings seem very unreal; here was something she recognized from her previous life. She pulled out the book that she had put in there as she was leaving her apartment to get in the limo. She set it to the side. She continued to look through the purse. All the usual stuff rolled around in the bottom. Brenda pulled out her lipstick. Her lips were already full and red on their own. From what she had seen in the mirror this morning, it didn't look like she would be using much makeup anymore. As she sat there, she decided that she needed to see the light. She had been asleep or unconscious all week during the day.

Suddenly, she missed the sun. For some reason, she was having trouble remembering how it felt on her skin. Brenda crossed the room to the window. She opened the drapes to expose a blind. She found the drawstring and pulled. It was cloudy and there were several large trees near the house. She stared out and realized that the rear of the house backed up to a set of woods. The clouds parted just enough to allow a shaft of light to fall through the window.

Brenda heard a loud hissing noise. She was startled to find that she was crouched on the other side of the room making that sound. The part of her brain that attacked Galen last night obviously didn't like the sun. Other than the fact that it seemed extraordinarily bright at this moment, there seemed to be no immediate danger. She braced herself and walked back over to the window as part of her screamed to run. The other more rational part of her knew how to close the blind. After she closed the drapes, she felt shaken. None of this had been a dream. She really had become a vampire. Not the kind of thing she had seen in the movies, but a real, living, breathing creature that hunted for its food.

The thought of having to kill to live was not an easy thought for her. Tears began to roll down her cheeks. Brenda sat down heavily in Galen's chair. This wasn't like ordering fried chicken or a steak. This wasn't even like having to go hunting. She had been hunting before. You killed it, you cleaned it, and then you cooked it. No, this was nothing like that. Now, you could have a conversation with dinner. Now, you actually talked to the dinner and it talked back. Playing with your food suddenly had a whole new meaning. She shook her head as tears streamed down her cheeks. She wanted to stop this kind of thinking.

Brenda looked around the room at the fine layer of white dust that covered everything. Her eyes settled on the fine taper candles in crystal holders on the credenza. Curiosity overcame her caution as she reached for the fancy looking box of wooden matches. If she didn't like the sunlight, how would she do with candles? She had always liked candlelight. She could remember all of the candles at church when she was a child. Carefully, she struck the match and it flared into life. The scent of sulfur assailed her nose. Quickly, she lit the first candle and blew out the match. She dropped the remainder into the ornate metal wastebasket. A gentle, vanilla scent rose into the air from the flame. She used the first to light the other six. The gentle glow didn't terrify her the way the direct sunlight had. Brenda felt a perverse pleasure in keeping the hungry little flames trapped as candles. She also felt a sample of the rage that the flames released. She imagined that she could feel their hunger. The candles started to remind her of church and mortal sins like suicide and murder. She discovered that she was crying harder.

Brenda picked up the book from her purse. She stared at the cover as if it held the answer to her questions. The cover was dark, tooled leather with a diary lock. Carefully, she slid the mechanism back and the lock clicked open. She rubbed her fingers slowly along the outside edge of the pages. Her tears had stopped, but they looked like they could return at a moment's notice. She thumbed to the halfway point and opened the book.

Hollowed out books had been a fad many years ago. She had kept this one because it was real leather and her mini nine-millimeter handgun fit perfectly. She lifted out the cold steel and felt the weight of it in her hand. She picked up the clip and stared at the top round with intense interest.

With one fluid move, the clip locked into place. The next sliding action made the weapon ready to fire. This was real. You pulled the trigger and you killed something. You didn't have to talk, seduce, or fight with this. You aim and squeeze. Brenda's eyes wandered loosely over the gun. It was strange how this made her feel calm. She was trying to make up her mind. It seemed so easy to solve her problems this way, but something Galen said kept haunting her thoughts.

He had told her that they could be killed, but it was not easy. What did he mean by it was not easy? She looked at the gaping hole she had ripped in the wall with Galen's body. Brenda could see the hole in the far wall where she had put his head. She remembered the blows that she had received. Nobody should be able to hit as hard as he did. She was in pain and moved very stiffly, but she should have broken bones.

If they could take that kind of damage what would a gun do? Could she really end this or just make matters worse? She had never shot a person before. She held the gun to her temple. Brenda could feel the coolness of the metal against her skin. All it would take was one little squeeze. She had read somewhere about somebody doing this and living. What if she didn't die? She had bought this gun for protection, what was it protecting?

Brenda looked at the hole in the wall again, and then she thought of David. She placed the gun over her heart. Again she felt the cold steel. Somehow, she knew that this wouldn't work. This just looked like it would be too painful. She put the barrel at her throat under her chin. This time a glimmer of determination crossed her face. She took several deep breaths in preparation.

Her eyes wandered down to her lipstick. It was so mundane and normal. The tissues in the purse, the keys to her door, the compact, these things were just so normal that she couldn't stand what she had become. Brenda could feel a flush rising in her cheeks. The tears began rolling again. She would have liked to have the chance to say good-bye to a few people. She realized that there was really no one who would miss her right away. Work would just mark her down as a no-show and replace her. She really didn't have anyone close to her in her life right now. Eventually, they would open her apartment when she didn't pay the rent. Brenda hadn't seen or even called her family in months. There were a few friends that would miss her, but no one who would go looking very far. She realized why Galen had chosen her. She was perfect for him to make disappear, just like David.

Brenda began to sweat as her hand began to shake. Abruptly, she put the barrel in her mouth and squeezed her eyes shut. The muscles in her arms flexed as both hands gripped the gun so tightly that the knuckles turned bone white. One little squeeze...

She felt the finger tighten. She could taste the metal and gun oil. As she bore down, her lips curled back from her teeth. Somewhere in the distance, she could hear a roaring sound. It rushed closer.

The shock of the blast threw her from the chair. Drywall and dust poured down from the hole blown into the ceiling. The noise deafened her in one ear. The heat from the powder burned lightly at the side of her head. Brenda opened her eyes expecting to see someone there. When she had pulled the trigger someone or something had ripped the gun from its fatal position. She closed her eyes and she could see who her savior was. It looked like her, but it was more like an animal.

Suddenly, Brenda understood. It didn't matter what she wanted. It didn't matter what she felt or thought. What Galen had done to her had given the part of her brain that held the will-to-survive-at-any-cost the final say in all things. She couldn't do this now or ever. She had no choice except to decide how she was going to survive.

Utterly defeated, she stood up and numbly dropped the gun to the desktop then walked out of the study, the lit candles completely forgotten. She headed back to the bedroom. She hoped that Galen would get home soon. He would feed her. She was a little hungry, but she no longer had the spirit to do anything but lie in bed.

Chapter Twenty Five

Michelle had brought over the letters of authorization that she had requested. It was nearly three and Maggie felt like she was closing in on answers. As if fate suddenly decided to be on her side again, Michael Lawson came through her part of the office with a needy look on his face.

"Everything okay, Michael?" Maggie asked.

"Yeah. Well no. I have a meeting in a few minutes and I also need to pickup some papers from a client today. I was looking for somebody reliable to send out to pick up the papers." Michael answered looking directly at Maggie.

"Do we have to have the papers in the office today?" Maggie's hopes rose.

"No, it's just that this guy is going on vacation for two weeks and I'm going to need his numbers before he gets back." Michael explained hoping she would volunteer.

"I'll make you a deal. I'm caught up here and I have a few errands to run. If I pick up your papers," she paused then continued, "how about you let me off the rest of the afternoon?" Maggie tried to look convincing.

"Sure. It's Friday. Here's the address and I'll see you on Monday. Oh, go ahead and go. He's waiting. Thanks Maggie." Michael agreed heartily.

"No problem, Michael." Maggie tried her best not to run for the door. She grabbed the letters and her purse. She didn't even shut down her terminal. Rob could fuss at her later about it.

On her way to the front door she stopped at Tina's desk. "Tina, I'm going to run an errand for Michael. I won't be back today."

Tina looked up from her screen, "Okay, I'll see you Monday. When are you going to explain all this Mircalla stuff to me?"

"I'll explain everything Monday, I hope. See ya." Maggie waved as she went out the front door and hurried to her car. The client's office was not far and it was in the same direction as Mr. Mircalla's address. She walked into the office, and to her relief, the papers were in a large, brown envelope waiting at the front desk. The receptionist looked up as she approached.

"I'm here to pick up some papers for Lawson Accounting." Maggie looked at the envelope as she spoke.

The woman behind the desk smiled and pointed. "There they are."

"Thanks. You have a nice weekend." Maggie picked up the envelope and turned towards the door.

"You too." The woman said as she looked back down at her screen.

Maggie tossed the envelope into the back seat and pulled out onto the street. Mr. Mircalla lived at the edge of town in an exclusive suburb. As Maggie turned onto his road, she admired the houses. They were spacious and set well back from the road. Maggie thought sarcastically about how tough it must be to have to drive from the house to the mailbox just to get your mail. There was the address that she was looking for. It happened to be at the end of the street, nearly hidden by bushes. She pulled into the drive. The house was similar to the others she had just passed, large and expensive. She parked in front of the house. Her faded red two-door vehicle looked somewhat conspicuously out of place.

She picked up the letters that she had brought with her and suddenly realized that she had no idea what she was doing. She began talking out loud to herself. "Maggie. What do you think you are doing? This guy is going to think you're a nut case. He's going to have you arrested. I can't wait to call Michael from jail and tell him I got busted hassling a major client. That will be nice."

Maggie sat there for a couple of minutes talking herself out of talking to him. All she had to do was wait for Monday. She started the car and put it in gear. She didn't pull away.

"No, damn it!" Maggie exclaimed to herself as she slammed it back into park. She gritted her teeth and got out of the car. There were no signs of life in the house. The windows were all dark with the blinds closed. Maggie walked up to the door and rang the bell. She fidgeted about nervously. She had no idea what she was going to say to this man when he opened the door. She still had no real idea why she was here. Perhaps it was closure. Her ex-husband really hadn't cared that a couple of her friends had disappeared so she never finished out her feelings. Now, maybe, she would be able to put this to rest. This was really the last thing left hanging in her mind from before she got married. With great resolution, she rang the bell again. She was going to get her answers today. She hoped.

Brenda had been lying on the bed staring at the ceiling when she heard a car pull up out front. She lay there and stared blankly at the ceiling not caring about anything. The car started again. Somewhere in her defeated mind, something took a little interest in the unusual sounds from the outside world. The only external sign of interest was that she allowed her head to fall to the side facing the sounds. The car engine stopped again. After what seemed to be an eternity, she heard a car door slam shut. She closed her eyes.

The doorbell rang. Brenda's eyes ripped open. She lay there in a sudden state of awareness. Her eyes darted from side to side as her breathing deepened. The bell rang again. Brenda sat up and sighed deeply. "If somebody is trying to sell something, they're going to regret stopping at this house."

Maggie had begun to lose her nerve again. She had rung the bell four times and no one had answered. She rang the bell one last time. A moment later, she heard someone inside at the door, working the lock. She steeled herself. He was going to open that door and she was going to have to go through with this. The door opened slowly. At first, she didn't see anyone.

"May I help you?" A woman's voice came from inside the hallway.

Maggie was stunned to see a young woman at the door. She expected almost anything but a barefoot woman to open the door. "Is Mr. Mircalla in?" Maggie ventured taking a step back.

"No, he had an errand to run. Can I help you?" The young woman responded.

The steam blew out of Maggie's sails. He wasn't even home. Maggie dropped the official tone and began explaining, "I'm sorry to disturb you. I'm Maggie DeVane. I'm with Lawson Accounting. I just had some papers for Mr. Mircalla to sign. I can come back later."

Maggie moved her hands around like a nervous five year old as she started backing down the steps. Brenda was now fully awake with conflicting wants. She could hear the blood moving through this woman's veins. She could even smell the woman's disappointment and nervousness. The woman was lying and Brenda's hunger and curiosity were both piqued.

"He'll be back soon. If you don't mind waiting, you can come in." Brenda said as she opened the door wider. She could smell the woman's mood change from defeat to optimism.

"I don't mind waiting. Thank you very much." Maggie said with renewed determination.

Brenda stepped back deeper in the hallway allowing Maggie to enter. "Just have a seat in the room to the left."

"Okay, thanks." Maggie walked into the sitting room. It was sparsely, but nicely furnished. Maggie sat down on the couch and looked up at Brenda standing in the doorway.

"I'm going to get a glass of ice tea. Can I get you one?" Brenda offered.

"Yes, please. It is a little warm out there today." Maggie replied politely.

Brenda disappeared and left Maggie to look around. There wasn't a lot to look over. The room had been tastefully decorated in earth tones with a blue and red paisley pattern on the couch and the two side chairs. The table was an oblong brass and glass, all new. Somehow, Maggie had figured on antiques and the cluttered Victorian look. She certainly didn't expect an athletic young woman to answer the door.

"This is just great. I'm hear to ask him about an old girlfriend while his new girlfriend is sitting here." Maggie muttered to herself.

Brenda filled the glasses with tea as she played with possibilities. Galen's accountant made house calls. This meant that he had real money. She knew that she would have to depend on Galen for a while. Sooner or later, she would find a way to get even with him.   Revenge through his money was as good as any other way.   Brenda wiped her forehead.   She was sweating slightly.   Her senses felt as if they had shifted into a higher gear.   It might be fun just to play with this woman for a little while.   She picked up the full glasses and walked lightly back to the sitting room.

"Here we go."   Brenda announced as she entered the room.

"Thank you."   Maggie replied as she took a sip.

As they both put their glasses down, Brenda asked, "How long have you been Galen's accountant?"

"Not long.   He transferred some of his business to our firm a few weeks ago."   Maggie replied trying to sound conversational.

Brenda fixated on the word "some".   This meant he had enough money in "some" of his business for an accountant to make house calls.   Brenda was at a loss as to how to find out how much.   While she was close to this woman, she could sense her fairly well, but last night followed by this morning's mishap had dulled her new abilities to the point that she couldn't hear anything more than just a few feet away.

"What did you say your name was again?"   Brenda couldn't think of anything else to say.

"Margaret DeVane, but everybody calls me Maggie."   Maggie smiled at the woman.

"I'm Brenda, I'm a ..ah .. friend of Galen's."   She said while extending her hand.

"Pleased to meet you." replied Maggie as she lightly shook Brenda's cool hand. Maggie's eyes were adjusting to the dim light inside. As she pulled her hand back from the greeting she could see the fresh lump on Brenda's forehead. She also seemed to be favoring her ribs.

"I don't mean to intrude, but are you okay?" Maggie couldn't help but ask.

Brenda self-consciously touched the bump on her forehead. It was a lot smaller than it had been earlier, but it must still be noticeable. Brenda realized that she hadn't even brushed her hair today.

"Oh, I'm fine. I was...," she paused for a moment, "in a car accident a few days ago. It wasn't bad, but I got banged up a little. Galen is letting me stay here for a while." Lying to a mere human seemed to come easily. Brenda could tell that she was still on guard. Touching her hand had confirmed that Maggie was here for something more than getting papers signed. There was something very determined about the woman.

The conversation didn't move smoothly for either of them. Awkward silence had so far dominated the conversation. Both of them were suspicious of the other. Brenda took the lead again. "How long have you known Galen?"

Maggie's jealous girlfriend alarm system began raising red flags. This Brenda was sitting too close and was looking at her with too much interest. Maggie began to feel uncomfortable under the scrutiny.

"I don't know him." She blurted out then continued more slowly, "I mean, I saw him at a company dinner. I was already coming out this way and just thought I would drop by."

Maggie was starting to look like she was going to leave. Brenda kept trying to keep her attention. Brenda's breathing began to deepen slightly. She could just begin to taste Maggie slightly through the air. She was very healthy.

"Relax, honey." Brenda said leaning back in her chair trying a new tactic. "I mean does he do a lot of business with your firm?"

Maggie relaxed slightly and said, "Not me personally, but our firm handles several domestic accounts for Mr. Mircalla."

"Really. I guess it takes a special kind of person to keep up with all those numbers and stuff." Brenda smiled and cocked her head to one side as she talked.

Maggie smiled. Brenda was a showpiece, looked good, not too brainy. She'll grow out of it. "Not really, it is like anything else. It just takes practice. Once you get used to the laws and the procedures it really isn't all that bad." Maggie relaxed a little more as she talked.

"I guess that you can get used to almost anything." Brenda said almost to herself.

"I guess so." Maggie agreed as she raised her eyebrows. Brenda must have been hit in the head pretty hard.

Brenda took a deep breath. This woman would taste strong yet sweet. She could get used to this feeling. "Have you been an accountant long?"

"I guess about seven years now. I just started back with Lawson's. I worked for them five years ago. Then I got married." Maggie's eyes rolled slightly at her last statement.

Galen said to only look for the ones that could disappear. "Do you have any children?"

"No, thank goodness. I just got a divorce a couple of months ago." Maggie answered wryly.

"I'm sorry to hear that." Brenda said, as she looked sad for her. She had no one right now.

"Don't be. Some things just don't work out. It feels good to be out on my own again." Maggie relaxed a little more into the girl talk.

Brenda began to enjoy the game. She began to understand Galen a little better now. "Have you been here long?" Brenda inquired next.

"No, I just moved here." Maggie shook her head. "I mean, I just moved back here. I lived here in town until I got married. I figured, I would move back and start over." There was still something strange about Brenda that bothered Maggie.

"Was Galen a client five years ago?" Brenda swung back to money. She ran her fingers through her hair.

"No, but it turns out we both had a friend in common back then. I was kinda hoping that he and I could talk about her." Maggie felt that she was getting too close to the real topic and reason for her surprise visit.

Brenda made up her mind at that comment. Galen wouldn't have human friends. Judging by this woman's age, her friend was most likely dead. She had been killed to feed Galen. It was Friday, no children, and no one at home. He had said to find the ones that wouldn't be missed. This one wouldn't be missed for several days and was a threat. Brenda was a little amazed at that thought. She, apparently, had begun getting used to these enhanced abilities. Galen also said if they were ever caught they would die horribly. Brenda asked, "Does your friend still live here in town?"

"No, she disappeared and was then found dead. I don't think anyone has had a chance to talk to Galen about what all happened." Maggie was starting to fidget. She did not want to stay on this topic with Brenda.

"That's a shame." Brenda said looking truly concerned as she finished the thought in her head, "That's a shame. I guess that you will get to do the same thing. This woman will taste strong and sweet."

CHAPTER TWENTY SIX

Maggie may have been relaxing a little, but Brenda's strange reactions and the tone in her voice kept Maggie from feeling comfortable. Right now, Brenda looked like she was trying desperately to make up her mind. Maggie decided that she would wait a few more minutes, and then she would leave. She would see Galen on Monday like they had already planned.

"Did you find out what happened to your friend?" Brenda asked to keep Maggie talking.

"The police said that her ex-boy friend kidnapped her and killed her. It was in the newspapers here. It was all very tragic." Maggie continued to fidget with the folder she had the papers in.

Watching Maggie intently, Brenda continued the verbal engagement. "That's terrible. Does anybody know why he did it?"

Maggie hadn't really planned to have this conversation yet, but Brenda seemed to be hanging on every word. It was hard not to talk to someone who listened well even if they made you a little uncomfortable.

"The police put it down as a murder/suicide. They said he was jealous and well that's what they said happened." Maggie shook her head sadly.

"Did you know the boy friend?" asked Brenda staring into Maggie's eyes.

"Yes, yes I did. We all went to high school together. I guess that's what makes all of this so hard to get over. I saw Galen at the company dinner and I knew that he had to be the same man that Jean, the woman who disappeared, had met." Maggie put the folder down and folded her hands into her lap.

Brenda was putting the story together very quickly. Galen had fed twice that trip. Galen must have taken Jean the same way he had taken her. The boy friend must have been a bonus. Brenda knew how to set up a man for feeding. David had been proof that even if you didn't know what you were doing you could dangle sex in front of a man and he would go for it. Brenda was feeling stronger just thinking about feeding. She had thrown Galen around like a rag doll. She wondered if she could do the same with this woman. If she couldn't seduce her, she could overpower her.

Brenda's intense gaze finally got the best of Maggie's resolve to see Galen. Maggie looked at her watch then looked back to Brenda. She still had that slightly confused look of concentration on her face.

"Look, it's starting to get late and I still have some errands to run. I'll just leave these with you and Galen can give me a call if he has any questions." Maggie picked up the folder and handed it to Brenda. They both stood up in unison.

"Please, don't go. I'm sure that Galen will be back any minute. I know he would hate to miss meeting you." Brenda looked pleading.

Maggie had already made up her mind to get out of there. Somewhere in the back of her head, something didn't feel right. She wasn't sure what and suddenly she didn't care to find out.

"No. Really, I've got to get moving before I get caught in rush hour traffic." Maggie stepped towards the door. She saw all the confusion leave Brenda. A weird look of determination now dominated her face.

"No. I think that you're going to stay here with me." Brenda's voice was now husky and rigid.

"What?" Maggie tried to edge to the doorway as quickly as possible without running.

Brenda debated for just a moment before the beast pushed its way to the front in her mind. It was hurt and it wanted to feed. A feeding would help the healing. After the attack on Galen, it was confident it could handle this human. After all, she was merely prey.

Maggie saw Brenda's eyes narrow. She got scared at this point. The woman was nuts. Maggie leaned backwards out of instinct. She barely saw the slap coming. Brenda moved faster than

212

anything she'd ever seen before. The impact spun her on her feet. Maggie saw lights swirling in front of her eyes. Before she could recover, she felt strong hands on her shoulders. Brenda yanked her around face to face. Maggie couldn't even get her hands up before she was shoved with tremendous force down onto the couch.

The smell of Maggie's shock and fear pushed the feeding instinct in Brenda over the edge. Putting one hand on Maggie's shoulder and grabbing her hair with the other, Brenda abruptly exposed Maggie's neck. With a great hiss, Brenda reared back then lunged for the exposed flesh. Brenda's chest exploded in pain as Maggie's knee smashed into the damaged area. All of the air rushed from Brenda's lungs as she doubled over in agony.

"Get off me you crazy bitch!" Maggie screamed at Brenda as she fell back. Maggie raised her leg and kicked Brenda in the center of the chest as hard as she could to clear the path to the door. As the shoe made contact with another damaged area, Brenda was hurled backwards onto the table. The safety glass disintegrated into thousands of gem-like pieces. The cascade of glass sounded like a crystal waterfall as it crashed down around Brenda's body. The sound that roared like a wounded great cat shocked them both as it escaped Brenda's lips.

The movement of Brenda trying to sit up broke the momentary paralysis that held Maggie. She bolted around the corner and ran towards the door. Maggie grabbed the handle. It wouldn't turn. Maggie scrambled at the locks. She screamed as a pair of arms tore through the wall grasping for her. A hand locked onto her arm like a vice. Maggie struggled wildly to get loose. She pulled as hard as she could, but she couldn't break the grip. The drywall flying out of the hole made the arms look an unearthly white.

"Let go! Damn you!" Maggie screamed as she clawed at the hand.

The grip wouldn't break. In desperation, Maggie flung her whole body against the elbow side of the arm. An unreal howl from the wall tore into the air as the arm wrenched back, hyper-extending the elbow. Maggie pulled one more time. She was free. She ran back up the hall and turned down the next hall. There had to be another way to get out of here.

"Jesus Christ." Maggie cried out as she stumbled into the wreckage from the night before. There was a gaping hole in a wall and drywall scattered everywhere. The rest of the walls were either cracked or gouged. Maggie looked through the hole to see the melted candles still burning in an office. A noise behind her caused her to spin around. Brenda was right behind her. Her eyes flashed a hellish red. She still looked human, but she moved more like a prowling beast. Brenda leapt impossibly into the air, hurling at Maggie. In pure terror, Maggie threw her arms out in front of her. The impact drove her back through the hole into the study. Her hands accidentally collided with Brenda's midsection in the air. Brenda hit the ground like a wounded eagle.

Maggie shook her hands and stood up. Something in the corner of her eye caught her attention. There was a gun on the desk. Maggie grabbed it gun as she heard Brenda crawling through the hole. Maggie spun as Brenda lunged forward. Maggie squeezed off a single shot. The recoil jolted her arms lightly. The bullet ripped Brenda from her feet and slammed her to the ground backwards.

"Oh my God." gasped Maggie. Brenda lay still on the floor. "Oh my God." repeated Maggie as she covered her mouth in shock. She put the gun down on the desk and looked back at Brenda. She had not moved. Maggie stepped towards the felled woman. She couldn't tell if Brenda was breathing or not. A large red stain began creeping over the left shoulder. Maggie was almost in shock. She had never been involved in anything like this before. Maggie leaned over the body to see if she was still alive. She wasn't sure what to look for, but she felt compelled to help.

Before Maggie could say a thing, the right hand flew to her throat. The fingers tightened, trying hard to meet the thumb in the middle. Maggie gagged as she struggled to get loose. Again, she couldn't break that grip. Brenda was just too strong for Maggie. Since she couldn't get away, Maggie attacked Brenda. Brenda was now barely able to defend herself. Maggie could feel the conscious world slipping into nothing. She didn't have long before this crazy person choked her to death. As a last resort, Maggie smashed her knees down on Brenda's chest. The hand on Maggie's throat loosened, but didn't give up. Maggie smashed down again. This time the hand let go.

Maggie fell back then scrabbled to her feet. Brenda was bleeding badly. She just lay on the floor, moaning slightly. Maggie almost got closer again then changed her mind. The woman was deranged. She was also shot and losing a lot of blood.

Maggie screamed as Brenda sat up. Maggie grabbed the gun from the desk where she had set it down. She ran out of the door into the hallway and looked back into the hole. Brenda was not there. Maggie flattened out on the wall and edged towards the door. She found herself doing the same maneuvers that she had used with Rob and the water pistols. This time, she played for her life.

Brenda was having a great deal of difficulty finding Maggie. After this morning, she couldn't pick up the small sounds that would normally have led her directly to her prey. Maggie could see a faint shadow in the doorway. She gritted her teeth. She tried desperately to remember everything Rob had ever told her. She tried to calm down her breathing. Somehow, imagining that she held her water pistol seemed to help. Maggie could just barely hear the sound of Brenda stepping on a piece of paper somewhere near the door. It was now or never. Maggie spun into the doorway. Her sights centered, aimed at no one. Rob's teasing about where people hide swung her aim to the door side of the room as Brenda lunged forward.

Two shots rang out wildly before Brenda slammed into Maggie. The momentum carried them both across the hall where they crashed into the wall. They collapsed down into a tangled heap. Drywall dust flew up in to the air at the impact and began settling over the unmoving forms.

CHAPTER TWENTY SEVEN

There was a small, red car with a "Don't Laugh It's Paid For" bumper sticker on it in front of the house. A wave of anger and concern swept through Galen. It was too soon for Brenda to be near any human. She would attack. He should have pulled her heart out while he had the chance.

"Damn. This just isn't my freaking month." He said looking at the car. He admired Brenda's passions and strengths, but she had become trouble personified for him. The only thing he could do now was hope that she hadn't complicated things too much while he was out. He had already made all of the arrangements to leave, but he had planned on having a few more days.

Galen tapped his fingers impatiently on the steering wheel as he waited for the garage door to open. He parked hurriedly and ran to the back door, still locked. Galen took a deep breath as he put the key in the lock. So far, he couldn't hear anything coming from the inside. He opened the door and the scent of gunpowder and blood assailed his senses. Galen walked stiffly into the main area of the house. He stopped at the front door. The scent of a woman hung in the air here. There had obviously been a struggle at the door. A hole had been ripped in the wall from the parlor to the front entryway. Galen shook his head.

"Brenda, you are hell on the walls." He said through clenched teeth.

He saw a manila folder on the floor. Some damn fool had come to the house. The smell of gunpowder and blood were very powerful now. Galen knew the smell of *upir* blood. Brenda had been wounded. Carefully, Galen walked towards the study. He didn't know what to expect, but he wasn't going to underestimate Brenda's reactions again. He was still in a great deal of pain because of her. There against the wall lay a bloody heap.

It looked like Brenda had her victim trapped underneath her, but there was too much blood on the ground for a feeding and the air was not charged with energy. Galen could hear breathing from the pile of bodies, but he couldn't tell who was still alive. He touched Brenda. She was barely above room temperature. Tenderly, he gathered a hand full of her hair at her scalp. He rubbed it softly between his fingers.

After a deep breath, he lifted Brenda off the woman. The woman's arm dropped to the ground as he lifted. At the last possible second, Galen saw something dark in her hand, a glint of metal. He hurled himself backwards, flinging Brenda's body to the side.

As the hand and the butt of the gun hit the ground, the woman flinched. The resulting explosion shocked her awake. The inhuman scream caused her to begin crawling backwards down the hall away from the bone chilling sound.

Galen saw the hand drop. He saw the flash as his sensitive ears were pounded by the sound. The impact of the nine-millimeter bullet ripped into his thigh mid-leap. At this close range, the impact threw the leg backwards in the air causing him to crash face first to the ground. He hit hard, screaming in frustration. He had never had this bad a run of luck ever in his long life. In case she pulled the trigger again, he rolled back away from the corner. The severe wound in his leg burned ferociously with every move.

Galen rolled up to the wall and braced his still painful back against it. He was losing precious blood. Every drop weakened him further. He ripped the sleeve from his shirt then ripped a smaller piece off. He rolled the smaller piece up into a ball and stuffed into the hole. His entire body stiffened with the pain. There was no exit wound. That would mean more pain later. At least the bone didn't feel broken. Galen wrapped the shirtsleeve around his leg and tied it tight to keep the makeshift plug in place. He worked as fast as possible, but he could hear that it was already too late. He looked up into the eyes of the woman and the barrel of the gun.

The scream had stopped. Maggie looked at that end of the hall and she saw the blood spray on the wall. She could hear the ripping of cloth and the muffled sounds of something moving around on the floor. She walked back up the hall holding the gun military style in front of her. Whatever was around the corner was injured and she intended to keep it that way. She stopped at the corner. She set herself then spun out into the opening.

The only reason she didn't pull the trigger was that there was a man lying there. She expected a mountain lion or something like that from the sound. They locked eyes for over a minute, neither of them moving, neither of them even trying to think. Both of them simply waited to react. Galen was the first to lower his eyes.

"Before you shoot me again, can I ask you for your name?" He looked at his wound while he spoke. He knew perfectly good and well who she was. He wanted her to start talking and give him time to think.

That accent, that was Galen lying there. She recognized him now. Her head hurt and it was a little hard to think right now. Maggie had no intention of getting close to him after what Brenda had done. Maggie suddenly felt very formal. "Mr. Mircalla, my name is Margaret DeVane."

"If I may call you Maggie, I thought we were not going to meet until Monday." The expression on his face was as if they were having a normal conversation in a restaurant, not a blood-strewn hallway. Something about his calmness angered her.

"That's right you bastard, we were. Instead, I decided not to wait. You see - I wanted to talk to you about Jean's disappearance. So I took off from work, drove over here, and your little psycho bitch tries to tear my head off. I'm in no mood for any bullshit out of you." Maggie stayed in her stance as she spoke. Maggie was almost shocked at the harshness of her words.

Galen could see and feel that Maggie would pull the trigger at any provocation. The woman was rattled and very defensive. She must also be very hard to kill. Brenda was ample, mute evidence of that, hard to kill or not, she now posed a direct threat that he would have to deal with immediately. Galen's style was to set up the time, place, and conditions for confrontations. He always stacked the deck in his favor, always in full control. Right now, he wasn't in control and his opponent was unstable. Stalling was the best tactic.

"Please be careful with that," he paused, "and tell me what happened here. After all, it is my home." Galen looked around at the damage to illustrate his point.

She reset her stance then answered. "Look, all I know is I knock on the door and Brenda or whatever her name was let me in. We sat down in the parlor for a couple of minutes. You're not here so I decide to leave and she attacks me. What the hell is she? I shoot her and she still gets up."

Maggie wasn't breathing as hard now, but she wasn't going to drop her guard. Galen decided that he if he tried to mislead her, she would anger again, and continue shooting. He needed a couple of more minutes to regain enough strength to deal with her. He might as well try to see if the truth would be bizarre enough to break her down and make her vulnerable.

"I'm afraid that you have stumbled onto a secret of sorts. Brenda was trying to kill you because that is what she does." Galen explained calmly.

"What is she, some kind of professional hit man or something?" Maggie tightened up her stance again. This change to a lecture worried her, but she came here for answers and it looked like she might get them. Her head continued to clear a little more. The scene may be unreal, but she was in it this far. She was terrified, but very determined.

Galen remained careful at gunpoint. Maggie seemed willing to listen. She could hear anything she wanted. She wouldn't leave here alive. "I think or something would best describe what Brenda has become."

"What do you mean - become?" She asked as her head cocked to one side, her hair flattened by blood, drywall, and sweat.

"Let me put it this way, Brenda hungered and she was going to feed on you." Galen explained with a calm expression.

She stared hard into his eyes, trying to detect a lie. She couldn't see anything in their dark depths. "She's some kind of cannibal or something?" Maggie queried in disbelief.

"The proper term is *upir*, where I am from. Your movies would call her a vampire. I was helping her through the transition from human to *upir*." Galen still had a straight face.

Maggie grew angry at this, "Bullshit, you're lying." Then she added an after thought. "It's daylight."

"This is not some pathetic B-movie with creatures of the night bursting into flame or cringing at the sign of religious symbols. An *upir* is a living being, just like you are. And just like the human race, the *upir* must kill to live." Galen flinched slightly from the pain in his leg.

Maggie couldn't believe that she was being drawn into this type of conversation with someone she had just shot and now had at gunpoint. So long as he didn't move or try anything, she would let him babble on. Maybe, they were members of some weird cult and Jean had become mixed up with them.

"We don't kill to live." Maggie argued.

"I believe that the cattle, swine, fowl, and sheep of the world would successfully argue that humans most certainly enslave, and kill to survive." Galen debated.

"And Brenda eats people. Do you expect me to believe this?" Maggie almost relaxed the grip on the gun.

Galen shook his head. "No. I do not expect you to believe any of this. That is what is so nice today. People will not believe in anything. They do not believe their governments. They do not believe their religious leaders. They do not even believe the stories handed down from their ancestors. Folk stories, myths, and superstitions they are called today. This is the modern dark ages." Galen looked like he was enjoying this part of the lecture. As he talked, the expression on his face became excited attracting her attention. She paid attention to his words, not his hands. "Where everyone is disillusioned and so broken hearted that they do nothing about it. People today do not even believe in themselves. If you try to tell anyone what you have seen or heard today you will, at best, be ridiculed and humiliated, at worst, placed under psychiatric care. If you do not believe me then at least believe what you have seen."

A slight noise behind her reached her ears. She stared hard at Galen, then glanced down the other hallway, nothing there. Something about that was very wrong, but a ripping sound came from Galen's direction. Her eyes snapped back forward as she lost her footing. Galen had ripped up the carpeting and was literally yanking it from under her feet. The gun went off into the ceiling. The sound, in the hallway, was deafening. She desperately rolled to her back bringing the gun up only to have it slapped out of her hands. Galen already stood over her. Nobody moved that fast was the only thought she had time for before he grabbed her throat with both hands.

She heard the gun clatter to the ground in the doorway of the study. Galen growled in pain as he lifted her to her feet. He slapped her to the wall next to where Brenda had put him. Pain exploded in her back and the back of her head. She saw lights in front of her eyes again.

"You want to know what happened to Jean Talbot. I will be happy to tell you. I met her. I listened to her problems and desires. I granted her a release from her miserable life. The end of her life allowed me to continue mine. We must feed to survive. The fact that you remember makes you a threat to my survival. Fortunately for me and my kind, humans no longer believe in anything that does not fit into their very limited definition of reality." Galen's eyes blazed. "Your disappearance will be made so bizarre that no one will ever figure out what happened to you. Someone will come up with a story that will be completely fiction, but it will fit what they want to believe."

Maggie hung there completely limp as she tried to gather some strength.

"He's going to kill me." She understood that now. A chill overtook her as he talked. His face drew closer. Maggie could feel a lethargy creeping into her muscles. She didn't want to die like this. The popping sounds coming from her neck and spine told her that her feet were no longer on the ground. She tried to focus on his face. It was quite close now. She could feel his body pressing up against hers. Strangely, it felt more like a lover's embrace than that of a murderer. She still didn't want to die like this. A shock passed through her body as his lips touched the side of her neck. He must have moved his hands. Her hands were trapped between their bodies. With the back of her hand, she could feel the bandage she saw him apply to his thigh. She tried to focus on the hand. Eventually, Maggie turned her hand over. She could feel the makeshift patch in his leg with her thumb. Waves of arousal swept down her body. He had set her down and one hand explored her body. The warmth gathering between her legs seemed to give her strength. The tempo of his breathing was rising. Had they been in the act of making love, his finish would have been eminent. They weren't making love. She knew it was time to choose whether to live or die.

Maggie put her thumb directly over the patch. She didn't want to die like this. She felt his weight shift and his breath against her skin. She was both very warm and very cold now. She could feel the lips lock onto the skin. She shoved her thumb as hard as possible into the wound in his leg.

The sound of the scream was unearthly, like a soul being rent in purgatory. The mist before her eyes seemed to explode. Feeling rushed back into her limbs. She applied more pressure. The patch gave way. She shoved the wadding deeper into his leg. Her thumb sank into his flesh up to the joint. His arms flung outward and his head went backwards as if he were being electrocuted. The scream continued to the breaking point of Maggie's nerves.

Abruptly, Galen's head snapped back down. His eyes blazed with pain and hatred. With a deep growl, he grabbed her shoulders and flung her through the open doorway of the study. She slammed into the desk and sprawled across it. Papers flew up in a cloud. Maggie hurt everywhere, but she knew she had to keep moving or she would be dead in an instant. She struggled to her feet and looked for Galen. He stood in the doorway. His face, the perfect picture of ultimate pain as he pulled the cloth from the profusely bleeding wound.

Maggie looked wildly around the room. She couldn't see the gun, but she did see a piece of paper burning on the credenza. It must have landed on the lit candles. Maggie ran to the flame and grabbed a handful of the scattered papers. She held them over the candles for a moment until the edges flared up. She rushed Galen with the ball of flame held before her.

"Burn! You son of a bitch!" Maggie shrieked as she slammed the burning paper into Galen's face. With the cry of a frightened beast, he tried to leap away. The damage to his leg pulled him up short and he rolled to the floor. Swatting at the flames like a great cat, he slapped them out. He rose to his feet. His precious blood ran freely from his body.

The expression on his face was no longer human. He was going to grant her a release from the pain of being alive by feeding. Now, he was simply going to enjoy ripping her apart. He didn't want to take her blood. He wanted to send it to hell for the devils to take. An orange glow and crackling sound forced him to crouch in alarm. His leg failed and he dropped to one knee.

Galen's struggle with the fire in the hall gave Maggie precious moments that she needed desperately. She looked around the room for the gun or anything else she could use. He had seemed terrified of the fire. Maggie ran to the far side of the room and pulled the drapery down. She balled it up and used the rod to carry it. As she came around the desk with her burden she saw the gun on the floor. The papers behind her had caught the flames and the room had begun to burn. Smoke filled the whole area quickly. It was getting hot and hard to see. This whole place would be coming down. She had to make a run for it quickly. She picked up the gun and stuck it in her waistband. She held the curtain over the spreading fire until it was ablaze.

As she burst from the room, Galen was in the center of the hall on one knee. She hurled the drapery from her like a fisherman casting a net. Galen struggled to his feet as the flaming material fanned out and covered him. As he disappeared behind the flames and smoke, she aimed for the center of the flaming mass and pulled the trigger. Shot after shot ripped through anything in the hallway until the gun stopped responding. As a last act of frustration, she threw the gun down the hallway with a growl of her own.

"You son of a bitch!" She said as she turned and walked away. The tears streaming down her face and the smoke made it hard to see. She found her way back to the front door. Her purse and the papers she had used as a pretense were still in the hall where she had dropped them. She picked up the purse and put the strap over her shoulder. She gathered up the papers. The sound of the breaking glass came from the direction of the fire. Calmly, she undid the locks on the door, as the smoke grew thicker.

She walked out into the front yard and turned to look at the house. She could see the flames through a front window. She turned and walked calmly to her car. Her keys were still in the side pocket of her purse. She got in her car, looked in the rear view mirror and buttoned her blouse. She started the car and pulled away without looking back.

Epilogue

Maggie drove home, completely numb. She made it inside and sank down onto the edge of her bed. That was the last thing she remembered.

Her back hurt, there was a bump on the back of her head, and her feet were cold. She lie on the bed fully dressed in clothes that smelled of smoke. The clock on the nightstand said 2:00. She didn't want to believe it. Maggie sat up and hurt everywhere. She managed to stand up and get undressed at the foot of the bed. Nude, she walked to the bathroom, and turned on the shower. Once the water was just right, she sat down in the tub, and let the water cascade over her. She didn't move again until the hot water began to run cold.

Maggie stretched a little while she dried off. A few small bruises had already begun to show on her back and neck. She didn't seem to care. She pulled a robe out of the closet and put it on. She walked out to the living room. The box of mementos sat on the bottom shelf of the bookcase. She pulled it out and sat down on the couch. She picked up the yellowed newspaper clippings. She didn't read them. They weren't true. They were accurate about the fact that two people were dead. The rest of the articles just made the facts fit a story that could be believed. Galen had been right. The facts had been created to cover the basics. The rest was simply ignored.

"Good-bye guys. Rest in peace." Maggie said as she nodded her head in relief. She kissed each article as she folded them up and put them on the bottom of the box. She stood up and carried the box back to the bookcase. As she passed the curio cabinet, she stopped and peered inside the glass.

"I know, take it easy. That's good advice, Saturday." She said to the gnome leaning against his tree stump. She walked back to the bedroom and climbed under the covers this time.

The next time she looked at the clock, it said 11:00. Maggie sat up and yawned. She was still a little sore, but she felt better. After her shower, she sat down with the newspaper and a pastry. The coffee was still brewing. In the local news section, there was an article about a house fire in the suburbs. The house had been badly burned before the fire department had arrived. There were no bodies found inside. Maggie figured that they probably turned to dust or melted away. The article also said the police had been unable to locate the owner yet.

Maggie smiled to herself. "Go ahead, keep looking." She knew that it was over, but she kept the door locked all day. Galen had been right about another thing. Who could she tell? Who would believe her? Even if she did come forward, what would the authorities do? Charge her with arson? Maggie decided to pretend the world was the same place it had been Friday morning. She would return to her world of debits, credits, and depreciation on Monday. However, she would make sure that someone else handled the Mircalla account. She just didn't want to know anymore.

Monday morning appeared almost surrealistic in how normal it was. Maggie felt pretty good when she woke up. She had breakfast and dressed for work like she did every Monday. She was surprised that even the bruises on her body had already faded substantially. As she looked in the mirror, she realized that she now carried with her a dark truth, a secret that no one would ever believe. She would never be able to see the world the same way again, but she would try.

The business world hummed into action as if everything were right in the world. Michael Lawson came through around mid-morning looking slightly distressed. He told Maggie and the rest of the gang that an accounting firm in Austria had faxed over a letter of authorization signed by Mr. Mircalla dated yesterday. It seemed that he had to go overseas on urgent business and wouldn't be back this year. Please forward his records to the address at the bottom of the page. Tina, Rob, and Morley all became very concerned as Maggie turned deathly pale and appeared faint. She explained that she must have been coming down with the flu.

Printed in the United States
107464LV00003B/68/A